Hip Arthroscopy

Editor

F. WINSTON GWATHMEY

CLINICS IN
SPORTS MEDICINE

www.sportsmed.theclinics.com

Consulting Editor
MARK D. MILLER

July 2016 • Volume 35 • Number 3

ELSEVIER

1600 John F. Kennedy Boulevard • Suite 1800 • Philadelphia, Pennsylvania, 19103-2899

http://www.theclinics.com

CLINICS IN SPORTS MEDICINE Volume 35, Number 3
July 2016 ISSN 0278-5919, ISBN-13: 978-0-323-44856-7

Editor: Jennifer Flynn-Briggs
Developmental Editor: Donald Mumford

Clinics in Sports Medicine (ISSN 0278-5919) is published quarterly by Elsevier Inc., 360 Park Avenue South, New York, NY 10010-1710. Months of issue are January, April, July, and October. Business and Editorial Offices: 1600 John F. Kennedy Blvd., Ste. 1800, Philadelphia, PA 19103-2899. Customer Service Office: 3251 Riverport Lane, Maryland Heights, MO 63043. Periodicals postage paid at New York, NY and additional mailing offices. Subscription prices are $340.00 per year (US individuals), $597.00 per year (US institutions), $100.00 per year (US students), $385.00 per year (Canadian individuals), $737.00 per year (Canadian institutions), $235.00 (Canadian students), $470.00 per year (foreign individuals), $737.00 per year (foreign institutions), and $235.00 per year (foreign students). Foreign air speed delivery is included in all *Clinics* subscription prices. All prices are subject to change without notice. **POSTMASTER:** Send address changes to *Clinics in Sports Medicine*, Elsevier Health Sciences Division, Subscription Customer Service, 3251 Riverport Lane, Maryland Heights, MO 63043. Customer Service (orders, claims, online, change of address): Elsevier Health Sciences Division, Subscription Customer Service, 3251 Riverport Lane, Maryland Heights, MO 63043. **Tel: 1-800-654-2452 (U.S. and Canada); 314-447-8871 (outside U.S. and Canada). Fax: 314-447-8029. E-mail: journalscustomerservice-usa@elsevier.com (for print support); journalsonlinesupport-usa@elsevier.com (for online support).**

Reprints. For copies of 100 or more of articles in this publication, please contact the Commercial Reprints Department, Elsevier Inc., 360 Park Avenue South, New York, NY 10010-1710. Tel.: 212-633-3874; Fax: 212-633-3820; E-mail: reprints@elsevier.com.

Clinics in Sports Medicine is covered in *MEDLINE/PubMed (Index Medicus) Current Contents/Clinical Medicine, Excerpta Medica,* and *ISI/Biomed.*

Contributors

CONSULTING EDITOR

MARK D. MILLER, MD
S. Ward Casscells Professor; Head, Division of Sports Medicine, Department of
Orthopaedic Surgery, University of Virginia; Team Physician, James Madison University
Director, Miller Review Course, Charlottesville, Virginia

EDITOR

F. WINSTON GWATHMEY, MD
Assistant Professor, Department of Orthopaedic Surgery, University of Virginia,
Charlottesville, Virginia

AUTHORS

CHRISTIAN N. ANDERSON, MD
Tennessee Orthopaedic Alliance, The Lipscomb Clinic, Saint Thomas West Hospital,
Nashville, Tennessee

ASHEESH BEDI, MD
Chief, Sports Medicine, Gehring Professor, Orthopaedic Surgery, MedSport, University of
Michigan, Ann Arbor, Michigan

MATTHEW TYRRELL BURRUS, MD
Resident Physician, Department of Orthopaedic Surgery, University of Virginia Health
System, Charlottesville, Virginia

JOURDAN M. CANCIENNE, MD
Resident Physician, Department of Orthopaedic Surgery, University of Virginia,
Charlottesville, Virginia

JAMES B. COWAN, MD
Resident Physician, Department of Orthopaedic Surgery, University of Michigan, Ann
Arbor, Michigan

BENJAMIN G. DOMB, MD
American Hip Institute, Westmont, Illinois; Hinsdale Orthopaedics, Hinsdale, Illinois

GUILLAUME D. DUMONT, MD
Assistant Professor, Department of Orthopaedic Surgery, University of South Carolina
School of Medicine, Columbia, South Carolina

MICHAEL A. GAUDIANI, BA
Department of Sports Medicine and Shoulder Service, Hospital for Special Surgery,
New York, New York

KIM GRAY, DPT
Physical Therapist, SMARTherapy, Washington Orthopaedics and Sports Medicine, Washington, DC

JUSTIN W. GRIFFIN, MD
Sports and Shoulder Surgery Fellow, Department of Orthopedic Surgery, Rush University Medical Center, Rush Medical College of Rush University, Chicago, Illinois

JAMIE GROSSMAN, MD
Research Fellow, Department of Orthopaedic Surgery, Lenox Hill Hospital, New York, New York

F. WINSTON GWATHMEY, MD
Assistant Professor, Department of Orthopaedic Surgery, University of Virginia, Charlottesville, Virginia

MICHAEL M. HADEED, MD
Resident Physician, Department of Orthopaedic Surgery, University of Virginia, Charlottesville, Virginia

JOSHUA D. HARRIS, MD
Assistant Professor, Department of Orthopedics and Sports Medicine, Houston Methodist Hospital Institute for Academic Medicine, Houston, Texas; Assistant Professor of Clinical Orthopedics, Weill Cornell Medical College, New York, New York

TIMOTHY J. JACKSON, MD
American Hip Institute, Westmont, Illinois; Orthopedic Medical Associates, Pasadena, California

ABDURRAHMAN KANDIL, MD
Orthopaedic Surgery Resident, Division of Sports Medicine, Department of Orthopaedic Surgery, University of Virginia Health System, Charlottesville, Virginia

ANTHONY KHOURY, MS
Hip Preservation Center, Baylor University Medical Center, Dallas, Texas

BENJAMIN KUHNS, MS
Division of Sports Medicine, Department of Orthopedic Surgery, Hip Preservation Center, Rush University Medical Center, Rush Medical College of Rush University, Chicago, Illinois

PAUL LEWIS, MD
Department of Radiology, University of Illinois Hospital and Health Services, Chicago, Illinois

ZACHARIAH S. LOGAN, MD
Department of Orthopaedics, Mayo Clinic Florida, Jacksonville, Florida

PHILIP MALLOY, MS, PT, SCS
Graduate Research Assistant and Doctoral Candidate, Department of Physical Therapy, Marquette University, Milwaukee, Wisconsin

HAL DAVID MARTIN, DO
Medical Director, Hip Preservation Center, Baylor University Medical Center, Dallas, Texas

SCOTT D. MARTIN, MD
Associate Professor, Orthopedic Surgery, Brigham and Women's Hospital/Harvard Medical School, Boston, Massachusetts

BRIAN A. MOSIER, MD
Sports Medicine Fellow, Orthopedic Surgery, Brigham and Women's Hospital/Harvard Medical School, Boston, Massachusetts

SHANE J. NHO, MD, MS
Division of Sports Medicine, Department of Orthopedic Surgery, Hip Preservation Center, Rush University Medical Center, Rush Medical College of Rush University, Chicago, Illinois

IAN JAMES PALMER, PhD
Hip Preservation Center, Baylor University Medical Center, Dallas, Texas

NOAH J. QUINLAN, MD
Orthopedic Surgery, Brigham and Women's Hospital/Harvard Medical School, Boston, Massachusetts

ANIL S. RANAWAT, MD
Associate Attending Orthopaedic Surgeon, Department of Sports Medicine and Shoulder Service, Hospital for Special Surgery, New York, New York

JOHN M. REDMOND, MD
Department of Orthopaedics, Mayo Clinic Florida, Jacksonville, Florida; American Hip Institute, Westmont, Illinois

MARC R. SAFRAN, MD
Professor, Department of Orthopaedic Surgery, Stanford University, Redwood City, California

RICARDO SCHRÖDER, PT
Hip Preservation Center, Baylor University Medical Center, Dallas, Texas

SARAH C. SPELSBERG, PA-C
Department of Orthopaedics, Mayo Clinic Florida, Jacksonville, Florida

ALEXANDER E. WEBER, MD
Division of Sports Medicine, Department of Orthopedic Surgery, Hip Preservation Center, Rush University Medical Center, Rush Medical College of Rush University, Chicago, Illinois

BRIAN C. WERNER, MD
Clinical Fellow, Department of Sports Medicine and Shoulder Service, Hospital for Special Surgery, New York, New York

ANDREW B. WOLFF, MD
Orthopaedic Surgeon, Department of Orthopedic Surgery, Washington Orthopaedics and Sports Medicine, Washington, DC

Contents

> Hip arthroscopy is a fast-growing and evolving field. Like knee and shoulder arthroscopy, hip arthroscopy began as a diagnostic procedure and then progressed to biopsy and resection of abnormalities. Subsequently, it has evolved to repair of various tissues and treatment of underlying causes. As the understanding of the hip joint and its associated pathophysiology grows, indications will continue to expand for this diagnostic and therapeutic modality. This article outlines the historic developments of hip arthroscopy, including advancements in instrumentation and techniques from the days of the first hip arthroscopies to the present day.

> Hip arthroscopy has experienced unprecedented growth in recent years and remains an area of booming technology and interest in orthopedic surgery. As understanding of the pathologic state of femoroacetabular impingement (FAI) has grown, imaging modalities have increased. Careful consideration of all bony and soft tissue structures in concert with physical examination findings in nonarthritic patients is necessary before any surgical intervention. This article summarizes the authors' approach to imaging in patients suspected of FAI, which facilitates careful patient selection and preoperative planning.

> The options for labral treatment are debridement, repair, and reconstruction. Debridement of labral tissue is indicated when there is peripheral tearing of the labrum that does not compromise the functionality of the labrum at its base or if the labrum is not playing an important role in the patient's pathology. Labral repair is performed when the base of the labrum is unstable at its attachment at the acetabular rim and the tissue is of otherwise good quality. Labral reconstruction is an option for labral tissue compromised beyond repair, segmental labral defect, or previous failed repair.

Disorders of the iliopsoas can be a significant source of groin pain in the athletic population. Commonly described pathologic conditions include iliopsoas bursitis, tendonitis, impingement, and snapping. The first-line treatment for iliopsoas disorders is typically conservative, including activity modification, physical therapy, nonsteroidal anti-inflammatory drugs, and corticosteroid injections. Surgical treatment can be considered if the patient fails conservative measures and typically involves arthroscopic lengthening of the musculotendinous unit and treatment of concomitant intra-articular abnormality. Tendon release has been described: in the central compartment, in the peripheral compartment, and at the lesser trochanter, with similar outcomes observed between the techniques.

Instability of the hip can manifest in a wide range of settings, with presenting symptoms including subtle discomfort at end range of motion or more dramatic dislocation of the joint. It can result from traumatic injury with dislocation or subluxation; atraumatic capsular laxity; structural bony abnormality, such as acetabular dysplasia; and iatrogenic injury. Initial treatment of the concentrically reduced joint often begins with physical therapy to strengthen dynamic stabilizers and to allow time for resolution of acute symptoms. Surgical treatment is aimed at repairing injured soft tissue structures, including static stabilizers, and addressing underlying bony structural deficiencies.

 Video content accompanies this article at http://www.sportsmed. theclinics.com.

Over the last decade, there have been significant advances in endoscopic techniques for peritrochanteric disorders of the hip. Endoscopic repair of gluteus medius and minimus tears has demonstrated good to excellent results in most patients who meet surgical indications with extremely low complication rates. Treatment of coxa saltans and other peritrochanteric disorders are also described, though the literature lacks sufficient evidence to guide treatment. As our understanding of peritrochanteric disorders evolves, endoscopic intervention will continue to progress with the development of improved technology to treat these disorders and ensure good outcomes.

Recent advances in understanding hip joint anatomy and biomechanics have contributed to improvement of diagnosis and treatment decisions for distal causes of deep gluteal syndrome (DGS). Ischiofemoral impingement and hamstrings syndrome are sources of posterior hip pain that can simulate symptoms of DGS. The combination of a comprehensive history and physical examination with imaging and ancillary testing are critical for diagnosis. Six key physical examination tests are described to differentiate distal versus proximal sources of extrapelvic posterior hip pain. Outcomes depend on patient compliance and the understanding of the entire anatomy, biomechanics, clinical presentation, and open versus endoscopic treatment options.

Although most patients have successful outcomes after hip arthroscopy, a minority of patients experience complications that may impact their recovery and long-term benefit. As most of these complications can be minimized by appropriate surgical technique, many tips have been recommended. Additionally, the reasons behind clinical failure postoperatively have been scrutinized, which include, most commonly, incomplete correction of osseous pathomorphology, underappreciated preexisting hip osteoarthritis, and/or an incorrect preoperative diagnosis. Meticulous preoperative planning, evaluation of advanced imaging studies, and proper patient selection will help to reduce the number of postoperative failures and increase the chance of a successful outcome following hip arthroscopy.

Adequate control of movement is essential for patients to return to unrestricted function after hip arthroscopic surgery. Mobility, muscle performance and stability, and neuromuscular control are vital aspects addressed in rehabilitation to help re-establish control of movement for function. Initial joint protection is a hallmark for all patients after hip arthroscopy to prevent intra-articular and extra-articular soft tissue irritation of healing tissues. It is essential to tailor exercises of each phase to patients' specific functional demands. Each phase of rehabilitation should be monitored so that patients are not advanced too quickly, which can lead to setbacks and delays in return to normal function.

CLINICS IN SPORTS MEDICINE

RELATED INTEREST

Orthopedic Clinics, April 2016 (Vol. 47, Issue 2)
Common Complications in Orthopedics
James H. Calandruccio, Benjamin J. Grear, Benjamin M. Mauck, Jeffrey R. Sawyer, Patrick C. Toy, and John C. Weinlein, *Editors*
Available at: http://www.orthopedic.theclinics.com/

THE CLINICS ARE AVAILABLE ONLINE!
Access your subscription at:
www.theclinics.com

Foreword

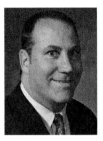

Mark D. Miller, MD
Consulting Editor

I am so proud of my junior partner, Dr Winston Gwathmey! I have considered myself a mentor of this excellent surgeon beginning with his rotation on my service as a medical student. He excelled as a medical student, resident, and fellow, and we were excited to invite him back to UVA on faculty. There was only one catch…we needed a hip arthroscopist, and if he wanted to return, he needed to be that guy! Once he learned enough about hip arthroscopy to even determine if he was interested, he took on this skill with the enthusiasm and excellence for which he is known. He went out of his way to participate in as many hip arthroscopies as possible during his fellowship, even though that wasn't part of the existing curriculum. Dr Gwathmey then went on to complete additional training in hip arthroscopy with Dr Thomas Byrd in Nashville, and he is now a legitimate expert in hip arthroscopy—and we are very happy to have him as part of our team!

Dr Gwathmey has assembled an excellent group of hip arthroscopy masters to share their experience in this issue of *Clinics in Sports Medicine*. It covers the entire gambit of this relatively new field from past to future. Hip arthroscopy has expanded rapidly, and we should recognize these experts with gratitude for "riding the wave" of this rapidly expanding area. Congratulations to Winston and sincere thanks to all who participated in this excellent issue!

Mark D. Miller, MD
Division of Sports Medicine
Department of Orthopaedic Surgery
University of Virginia
400 Ray C. Hunt Drive, Suite 330
Charlottesville, VA 22908-0159, USA

E-mail address:
mdm3p@virginia.edu

Clin Sports Med 35 (2016) xiii
http://dx.doi.org/10.1016/j.csm.2016.04.002
0278-5919/16/$ – see front matter © 2016 Published by Elsevier Inc.
sportsmed.theclinics.com

Preface

Advances in Hip Arthroscopy

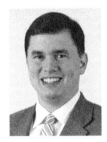

F. Winston Gwathmey, MD
Editor

Hip arthroscopy continues to evolve at a rapid rate. The expansion of indications and the advancement in technique over the past twenty years are truly remarkable. The arthroscope has provided invaluable insight into the pathophysiology of a variety of hip pathologies, including acetabular labral tears, femoroacetabular impingement, hip dysplasia, and gluteal tendon tears. It has allowed surgeons to effectively treat hip conditions that historically have required large open surgeries in a minimally invasive fashion with promising results. Hip arthroscopy continues to fuel new ideas and techniques to treat complex hip conditions.

As surgeons taking part of this dramatic evolution, we must realize that sometimes it is important to pause and consider where we came from, where we are, and where we are heading. This issue of *Clinics in Sports Medicine* is dedicated to hip arthroscopy, the current state of the procedure, and what is on the horizon. We are pleased to have brought together an outstanding group of authors who have contributed to the advancement of hip arthroscopy and share a passion and excitement for the future of the procedure.

Since it is essential to remember where we started, we open this issue with an excellent article by Drs Safran and Kandil on the history of hip arthroscopy. Dr Nho and his coauthors then detail the essential radiographic evaluation of a hip patient. We then considered the most common indications for hip arthroscopy and selected experts to author nine articles that cover the evaluation and treatment of these conditions comprehensively. Dr Bedi and his coauthors present critical cautionary information in their article on complications and risks of hip arthroscopy. We conclude the issue with Kim Gray and Phil Malloy's insight into the rehabilitation of a hip arthroscopy patient.

I sincerely thank all of the authors who contributed their expertise and effort to this issue. I would like to thank Drs Thomas Byrd and Scott Martin for sharing with me their

Clin Sports Med 35 (2016) xv–xvi
http://dx.doi.org/10.1016/j.csm.2016.04.001
0278-5919/16/$ – see front matter © 2016 Published by Elsevier Inc.

sportsmed.theclinics.com

expertise and enthusiasm for hip arthroscopy and giving me the tools to be a part of this exciting area of orthopaedic surgery.

F. Winston Gwathmey, MD
Department of Orthopaedic Surgery
University of Virginia
400 Ray C. Hunt Drive, Suite 330
Charlottesville, VA 22903, USA

E-mail address:
fwg7d@virginia.edu

Hip Arthroscopy
A Brief History

Abdurrahman Kandil, MD[a],*, Marc R. Safran, MD[b]

KEYWORDS

- Hip arthroscopy • History of hip arthroscopy • Evolution of hip arthroscopy
- Arthroscopy • Sports medicine

KEY POINTS

- Hip arthroscopy was first described by Michael S. Burman in 1931.
- The procedure was revisited in the mid-1970s, continues to become more popular, and now is one of the fastest growing areas within orthopedic surgery.
- Instrumentation has improved over the past 2 decades to better access the hip and treat intra-articular abnormalities.
- Indications continue to expand from treating hip abnormality to treating the underlying cause, and reconstructive procedures are being developed for damage that is not reparable.
- New complications are being encountered as utilization expands and more complex procedures performed.

INTRODUCTION AND KEY HISTORICAL DEVELOPMENTS

Hip arthroscopy was first described more than 80 years ago when Michael S. Burman performed the first recorded hip arthroscopy attempts on cadavers in 1931.[1] Hip arthroscopy was effectively deemed a futile procedure from the start by Burman, going so far as to say it is "manifestly impossible to insert a needle between the head of the femur and the acetabulum." However, although Burman had difficulty accessing the central compartment, he was able to visualize the peripheral compartment well.

Despite his ominous declaration, Burman made many important contributions to hip arthroscopy. First, he was the first to describe the paratrochanteric portal,

Disclosure Statement: Nothing to disclose. No commercial or financial conflicts of interest or any funding sources (A. Kandil). Nothing to disclose related to this article. Fellowship support: Össur, Breg, ConMed Linvatec, Smith and Nephew (M.R. Safran).
[a] Division of Sports Medicine, Department of Orthopaedic Surgery, University of Virginia Health System, Ray C. Hunt Drive, Charlottesville, VA 22908, USA; [b] Department of Orthopaedic Surgery, Stanford University, 450 Broadway Street, M/C6342, Redwood City, CA 94063, USA
* Corresponding author. 270 Riverbend Drive 4-C, Charlottesville, VA 22911.
E-mail address: Ak3ue@virginia.edu

which is close in proximity to the commonly used anterolateral portal today. He states, "The anterior para-trochanteric puncture is undoubtedly the best and is made slightly anterior to the greater trochanter along the course of the neck of the femur."

Second, he described the necessity of using long instruments to adequately traverse the generous soft tissue envelope surrounding the hip, an important feature in modern hip arthroscopy. He states, "A special long trochar [sic] with a correspondingly long telescope should thus be used for the hip joint." Current hip arthroscopy trays include extralong scopes as well as shortened bridge connectors to the camera that allows for a functionally greater working length while using regular knee arthroscopy scope lens.

Finally, although he used joint fluid distension and a 4-mm arthroscope (**Fig. 1**), there was no joint distraction, and visualization was limited. As a result, he could only visualize peripheral compartment structures that are easily viewed without traction, such as the femoral neck and head, but not the acetabular fossa, intraarticular labrum, and articular cartilage or ligamentum teres (**Fig. 2**). This finding later demonstrated the importance of joint distraction as a key component in obtaining adequate joint visualization, particularly of the central compartment.

In 1939, Kenji Takagi[2] reported the first clinical application of arthroscopy in the hip. He reported using hip arthroscopy as an adjunct tool in the treatment of a small 4-patient series of patients, including 2 Charcot joints, one case of tuberculous arthritis, and one case of septic arthritis.

Following this report by Takagi in Japan, there was no significant contribution to hip arthroscopy in the literature until the mid-1970s. In 1977, Richard Gross[3] reported the application of hip arthroscopy to pediatric disorders, including Legg-Calve-Perthes disease, slipped capital femoral epiphysis, congenital dislocation, and other pediatric conditions. Following this, the literature on hip arthroscopy expanded significantly, and numerous case series were being published in various journals. James Glick and Thomas Sampson contributed immensely to the literature in the 1980s and 1990s, discussing anatomy, indications, portal placement, and most notably, lateral positioning for hip arthroscopy.

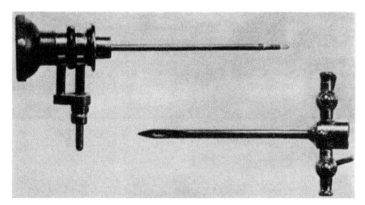

Fig. 1. Arthroscope and trocar used for joint arthroscopy in the landmark article by Michael S. Burman. The arthroscope divides into its 2 component parts: the upper is the telescope and the lower its sheath or trocar. (The illustration shows the arthroscope three-fourths actual size.) (*From* Burman M. Arthroscopy or the direct visualization of joints: an experimental cadaver study. J Bone Joint Surg 1931;13(4):671.)

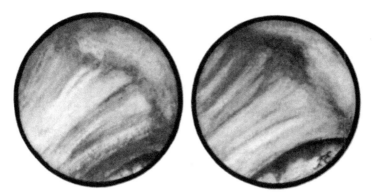

Fig. 2. Drawings of 2 views of the femoral neck using the "anterior paratrochanteric punc-ture." View obtained with "hip in external rotation, slight abduction, and neutral to flexion or extension…The neck of the femur with its ridings, the junction between head and neck, and a part of the head are seen. More of the superior and upper surface of the neck is shown." (*From* Burman M. Arthroscopy or the direct visualization of joints: an experimental cadaver study. J Bone Joint Surg 1931;13(4):673.)

In the mid-1990s, J.W. Thomas Byrd contributed greatly to numerous modifications in the hip arthroscopy technique and developed a hip arthroscopy study group that met between 1995 and 1998 at the Annual Arthroscopy Association of North America meetings that promoted the spread and exchange of ideas.

POSITIONING

Hip arthroscopy was initially described in the supine position (**Fig. 3**) and primarily used arthroscopic instruments designed for the knee and shoulder joints. In the late

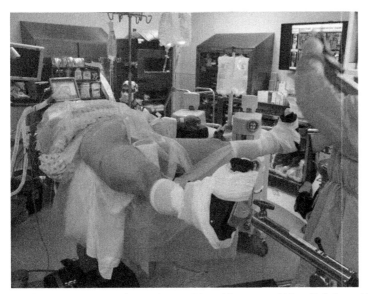

Fig. 3. Hip arthroscopy setup in the supine position. (*Courtesy of* Marc R. Safran, MD, Palo Alto, CA.)

1970s, reports began surfacing in literature about hip arthroscopy from the likes of Richard Gross, James Glick, and Thomas Sampson. Glick and Sampson helped pioneer the hip arthroscopy in the lateral decubitus position, whereas it had been previously done in the supine position.[4–6]

Glick reports that, in his early experience, he had difficulty getting access and adequate visualization of more than 40% of his patients using supine positioning on a fracture table, especially obese patients.[4] Glick and Sampson thought about a different way of getting into the hip joint and began experimenting with the lateral decubitus position. They described the technique in the lateral decubitus position with operative side upward. Skin traction straps were applied below the knee, and the operative limb was placed in a shoulder traction apparatus. The rationale for this position was that the soft tissue around the hip drooped away from the operative field, which helped accommodate shorter instruments. In addition, it also provided direct access into the joint, making it more accessible in obese patients.[4]

In the 1990s, J.W. Thomas Byrd[7] described modifications to supine patient positioning for improved visualization and increased safety. Byrd and colleagues[8] described techniques to minimize damage to the intra-articular structures when entering the hip joint in a supine position. He elegantly described the relative neurovascular anatomy to portals for hip arthroscopy. Some of his other contributions include describing the use of fluoroscopy and tactile sensation to decrease damage to the labrum.[9]

TRACTION

Visualization of the entire hip joint, including both the peripheral and the central compartments, has always been an area of interest and research in hip arthroscopy. Joint distension was used in early hip arthroscopy, but did not provide adequate visualization of the entire joint, particularly the area within the confines of the acetabulum (central compartment). As a result, early hip arthroscopy often managed disorders of the peripheral compartment of the hip (**Fig. 4**). The utilization of traction later became an extremely useful tool in improving visualization and expanding the role of hip arthroscopy in the management of hip disorders, particularly the structures of the central compartment: labrum, articular cartilage, and ligamentum teres (**Fig. 5**).

In the 1980s, Ejnar Eriksson and Lanny Johnson made major technique modifications in hip arthroscopy. In 1986, Eriksson and colleagues[10] studied the amount of force needed for adequate joint distraction to achieve sufficient visualization of the hip joint. The investigators found that the amount of force needed was reduced in an anesthetized patient experiencing muscle relaxation. They concluded that "in an anesthetized patient 300 Newtons (N) to 500 N was required, whereas up to 900 N was needed in an unanesthetized subject to achieve sufficient joint extension."

In the late 1980s, Henri Dorfmann and Thierry Boyer,[11,12] a pair of French rheumatologists, pioneered their own method of hip arthroscopy without distraction. This method was mainly used for visualization of the peripheral compartment. They posited that most hip abnormality was found in the peripheral compartment and can be adequately visualized without distraction. In reality, most synovial abnormality and loose bodies are evident in the peripheral compartment. Furthermore, Dorfman and Boyer contended that traction tightened the hip capsule, bringing the capsule closer to bone. Dienst and colleagues[13] more recently described the arthroscopic anatomy and systematic evaluation of the hip peripheral compartment.

For hip arthroscopy in the lateral position, Glick and Sampson used skin traction (25–50 pounds) to distract the hip joint and visualize the central compartment.[14] The

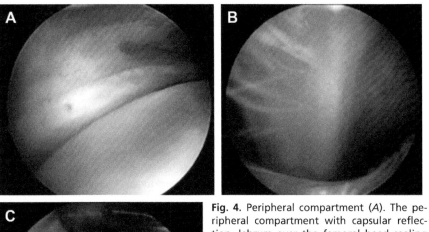

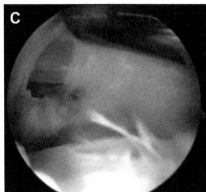

Fig. 4. Peripheral compartment (*A*). The peripheral compartment with capsular reflection, labrum over the femoral head sealing (*B*). Zona orbicularis over the femoral neck (*C*). Iliopsoas through cut in the capsule in the peripheral compartment. (*Courtesy of* Marc R. Safran, MD, Palo Alto, CA.)

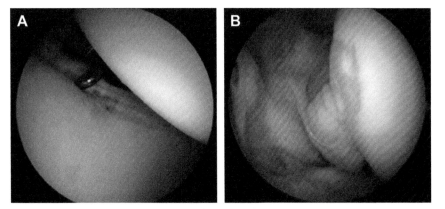

Fig. 5. Central compartment (*A*). Femoral head and acetabulum and labral tear at labral chondral junction anteriorly (*B*). Cotyloid fossa, big ligamentum teres, and femoral head with fibrocartilage near fovea. (*Courtesy of* Marc R. Safran, MD, Palo Alto, CA.)

hip joint inherently has negative pressure, resulting in resistance to distraction via the vacuum phenomenon. Central to the concept of traction is breaking the hip's suction seal by inserting a spinal needle and removing its stylet before applying traction.[11] This breaking of the suction seal decreases the amount of traction force necessary for distraction by allowing hip relaxation.

In the early days of hip arthroscopy, many patients underwent surgery on a fracture table, and most people still do today. However, as indications expanded and surgery was done on younger, more muscular patients, the need for modifications in positioning and equipment became apparent, leading to the development of hip-specific equipment to assist with traction. Various modifications were made over time to achieve traction, including a post for traction and countertraction for fracture tables. Tensiometers have also been used to gauge the amount of tension; however, they are not particularly accurate, and few people use them today. Hip-specific femoral distractors have been used for hip arthroscopy in either the lateral or the supine position. Some distractors improved the mechanical advantage to distract the hip away from the acetabular socket. Newer hip positioning systems allow even more control, including dynamic hip motion.

PORTALS

Portal placement has slowly evolved over the years (**Fig. 6**). The anterolateral portal was first described by Michael Burman in 1931.

In early hip arthroscopy, Glick described portals being made by placing a stab incision adjacent to a spinal needle, followed by placement of the arthroscopic cannula and trocar directed alongside the needle with the aid of an image intensifier.[15] The

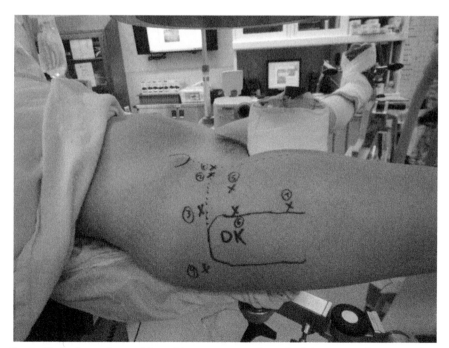

Fig. 6. Hip in the supine position with common portals marked. (*Courtesy of* Marc R. Safran, MD, Palo Alto, CA.)

capsule was incised in all directions, allowing for the placement and exchange of instruments without the need for a cannula. When cannulated instruments were developed, a nitinol guidewire was placed into the needle, and a cannulated trocar was placed over the nitinol guidewire, making it easier to replace instruments with one another.

Lanny Johnson[15] described the anatomic landmarks and proposed portal locations for hip arthroscopy. Byrd and Sweeney[8,16] also published on the anatomic landmarks for hip arthroscopy as well as relative relationships of the portals to the muscles they penetrated and neighboring neurovascular structures.

If bony landmarks are accurately marked, portal placement is relatively safe in hip arthroscopy. The superficial and palpable bony landmarks are the greater trochanter and anterior superior iliac spine. Deeper bony landmarks that are viewed fluoroscopically include the femoral neck and head.

Instruments passed through the anterolateral portal traverse the gluteus medius and minimus muscles. Instruments passed through the anterior portal traverse the sartorius and the rectus femoris muscles. The major nerve at risk with the anterior portal is the lateral femoral cutaneous nerve, approximately 15 mm from the portal. The major nerve at risk with the posterolateral portal is the sciatic nerve, which comes within 22 mm of the portal.[17]

INSTRUMENTATION

Michael Burman performed his first cadaveric dissections with a 4.0-mm-diameter arthroscope constructed by Reinhold Wappler, a size not too different from modern arthroscopes (see **Fig. 1**). Later in the 1970s, hip arthroscopy was performed with knee or shoulder instrumentation. Surgeons were unable to perform early hip arthroscopy consistently and completely with these instruments. Limitations included length and curvature differences between the hip and knee joints.

As the procedure became more popular, companies began to develop hip-specific instruments, including longer arthroscopes to make it easier to traverse the larger soft tissue envelope surrounding the hip. However, most hip arthroscopies are performed with standard length arthroscopes, but a shortened bridge connector between the sheath and camera/length/fluid connectors, making the working area of the arthroscope relatively longer. In addition, companies developed telescoping cannulas for the hip joint, which helped streamline the procedure by allowing the surgeon to maintain portal access throughout the surgical procedure. As with knee and shoulder equipment, there have been significant improvements in optical resolution, in addition to the development of hip-specific tools such as long arthroscopic graspers and straight, curved, and motorized shavers/burrs.

INDICATIONS

Hip arthroscopy was initially performed for simple intra-articular abnormalities, such as loose body removal in patients with mechanical hip symptoms or for irrigation and debridement in patients with infectious processes. In addition, early hip arthroscopy was a valuable diagnostic tool when other modalities failed to provide a definitive diagnosis.

Indications for hip arthroscopy have steadily expanded as familiarity with the procedure and the understanding of hip pathophysiology have evolved. The evolution of treatment has progressed from resection, such as partial labrectomy and debridement of articular cartilage, to more advanced procedures such as labral repair and reconstruction, microfracture, and autologous matrix-induced chondrogenesis for chondral lesions. Although early on the sequelae of injury and pathologic processes were being treated (labrum, chondral), now many techniques have been developed to treat the underlying cause (femoroacetabular impingement [FAI], instability), and these techniques continue to be refined and developed.

Indications for hip arthroscopy currently include management of labral tears, chondral injuries, adhesive capsulitis, instability, and synovial abnormality, among others (**Box 1**).[18] The most common diagnosis for hip arthroscopy today is FAI. Initially managed with an open surgical dislocation, FAI can now be adequately managed arthroscopically,[19] and studies comparing open versus arthroscopic management of FAI have shown similar outcomes, with less morbidity associated with the arthroscopic approach.[20]

In addition to intra-articular abnormality, there are extra-articular conditions that can be treated arthroscopically. These conditions include abnormality of the iliopsoas tendon and bursa, tensor fascia lata and trochanteric bursa, tight iliotibial band, and tears of the hip abductors. In addition, a subset of patients with hip dysplasia has associated intra-articular abnormality that may be addressed arthroscopically in the same setting as a periacetabular osteotomy (PAO) or even in lieu of a PAO.

FUTURE

Hip arthroscopy began as a diagnostic tool for unexplained hip abnormality as well as a therapeutic tool for simple procedures such as loose body removal and irrigation and debridement. Indications have expanded to include a large list of intra-articular and extra-articular hip processes. Focus has recently shifted to improving outcomes of arthroscopic hip surgery relative to open surgery, and there have been significant gains in this area.

As the understanding of hip pathophysiology continues to increase, hip arthroscopy will play an even greater role in the diagnosis and management of hip disorders. In the same light, indications for hip arthroscopy will continue to evolve with some indications becoming more popular and others going out of favor as real outcomes will

---

Box 1
Common indications for hip arthroscopy

Femoroacetabular impingement

Labral tears

Infection

Loose body removal

Degenerative disease

Chondral injury

Ruptured ligamentum teres

Instability

Adhesive capsulitis

Synovial disease

Iliotibial band abnormality

Hip abductor tears

Iliopsoas tendon abnormality

support or refute the use of hip arthroscopy in the management of these entities. Specialized hip instrumentation will continue to develop at a faster rate as the popularity of the procedure grows and industry sees a financial motivation to innovate in this area. A great deal of excitement lies in the future of hip arthroscopy, and the potential benefits for patients in this fast-growing field are very promising.

REFERENCES

1. Burman M. Arthroscopy or the direct visualization of joints: an experimental cadaver study. J Bone Joint Surg 1931;13(4):669–95.
2. Takagi K. The classic arthroscope. J Jap Orthop Assoc 1939; Clin Orthop Relat Res 1982;167:6–8.
3. Gross R. Arthroscopy in hip disorders in children. Orthop Rev 1977;6(9):43–9.
4. Glick JM, Sampson TG, Gordon BB, et al. Hip arthroscopy by the lateral approach. Arthroscopy 1987;3(1):4–12.
5. Glick JM. Hip arthroscopy using the lateral approach. Instr Course Lect 1988;37: 223–31.
6. Glick JM, Sampson TG. Hip arthroscopy by the lateral approach. In: McGinty J, Caspari R, Jackson R, et al, editors. Operative arthroscopy. 2nd edition. New York: Raven Press; 1995. p. 1079–90.
7. Byrd JW. Hip arthroscopy utilizing the supine position. Arthroscopy 1994;10: 275–80.
8. Byrd JW, Pappas JN, Pedley MJ. Hip arthroscopy: an anatomic study of portal placement and relationship to the extra-articular structures. Arthroscopy 1995; 11:418–23.
9. Byrd JW. Avoiding the labrum in hip arthroscopy. Arthroscopy 2000;16:770–3.
10. Eriksson E, Arvidsson I, Arvidsson H. Diagnostic and operative arthroscopy of the hip. Orthopedics 1986;9(2):169–76.
11. Dorfmann H, Boyer T, Henry P, et al. A simple approach to hip arthroscopy. Arthroscopy 1988;4(2):141–2.
12. Dorfmann H, Boyer T. Arthroscopy of the hip: 12 years of experience. Arthroscopy 1999;15(1):67–72.
13. Dienst M, Godde S, Seil R, et al. Hip arthroscopy without traction: in vivo anatomy of the peripheral hip joint cavity. Arthroscopy 2001;17:924–31.
14. Glick JM, Valone F III, Safran MR. Hip arthroscopy: from the beginning to the future—an innovator's perspective. Knee Surg Sports Traumatol Arthrosc 2014; 22:714–21.
15. Johnson L. Arthroscopic surgery principles and practice. St Louis (MO): CV Mosby; 1986.
16. Sweeney HJ. Arthroscopy of the hip. Anatomy and portals. Clin Sports Med 2001; 20:697–702.
17. Robertson WJ, Kelly BT. The safe zone for hip arthroscopy: a cadaveric assessment of central, peripheral, and lateral compartment portal placement. Arthroscopy 2008;24:1019–26.
18. Byrd JW. Hip arthroscopy. J Am Acad Orthop Surg 2006;14(7):433–44.
19. Sampson TG. Arthroscopic treatment of femoroacetabular impingement. Tech Orthop 2005;20:56–62.
20. Mardones R, Lara J, Donndorff A, et al. Surgical correction of "cam-type" femoroacetabular impingement: a cadaveric comparison of open versus arthroscopic debridement. Arthroscopy 2009;25:175–82.

Imaging in Hip Arthroscopy for Femoroacetabular Impingement

A Comprehensive Approach

Justin W. Griffin, MD[a], Alexander E. Weber, MD[b],
Benjamin Kuhns, MS[b], Paul Lewis, MD[c], Shane J. Nho, MD, MS[b],*

KEYWORDS

- Hip arthroscopy • Femoroacetabular impingement • Imaging • MRI • MRA
- Hip capsule • CT • Revision hip arthroscopy

KEY POINTS

- Plain radiographs, including anteroposterior pelvis, Dunn lateral, and false-profile view, are key in initial assessment of patients suspected of femoroacetabular impingement.
- Computed tomography scans rely less patient positioning and allow for accurate definition of the exact location and size of pincer-type and cam-type deformities, and can be particularly helpful in revision hip arthroscopy.
- Studies have shown high incidence of labral tears in asymptomatic patients, thus correlation between clinical and imaging findings is stressed.
- Systematic implementation of intraoperative fluoroscopy can assist in providing adequate acetabular and femoral decompression and avoid the most common cause of revision hip arthroscopy.

INTRODUCTION

The role of diagnostic imaging in femoroacetabular impingement (FAI) is to complement the clinical presentation and findings on physical examination. Diagnostic imaging provides objective information to the clinician, separate from confounding

[a] Department of Orthopedic Surgery, Rush University Medical Center, Rush Medical College of Rush University, 1611 West Harrison Street, Suite 300, Chicago, IL 60612, USA; [b] Division of Sports Medicine, Department of Orthopedic Surgery, Hip Preservation Center, Rush University Medical Center, Rush Medical College of Rush University, 1611 West Harrison Street, Suite 300, Chicago, IL 60612, USA; [c] Department of Radiology, University of Illinois Hospital and Health Services, 1740 West Taylor Street, MC 931, Chicago, IL 60612, USA
* Corresponding author. Division of Sports Medicine, Department of Orthopedic Surgery, Hip Preservation Center, Rush University Medical Center, 1611 West Harrison Street, Suite 300, Chicago, IL 60612.
E-mail address: nho.research@rushortho.com

Clin Sports Med 35 (2016) 331–344
http://dx.doi.org/10.1016/j.csm.2016.02.002
0278-5919/16/$ – see front matter © 2016 Elsevier Inc. All rights reserved.
sportsmed.theclinics.com

variables and unclear history. This can support or negate FAI among competing diagnoses. That said, abnormal femoral morphology and other findings consistent with FAI alone are not diagnostic for FAI if the corresponding clinical findings and/or symptoms are absent.[1] As a result, during initial work-up and preoperative planning, it is critical to choose the right diagnostic studies to answer the clinical questions at hand.

This article provides a comprehensive approach to imaging in FAI, from initial office-based radiographs to advanced preoperative 3-dimensional (3D) imaging. At any point imaging is used, it is important to evaluate the whole picture and consider pelvic joint abnormalities and muscular injuries that may mimic the symptoms or findings of FAI.

PLAIN RADIOGRAPHY

Plain radiographs play a key role in initial management of patients presenting with hip pain when FAI is suspected. Several options exist regarding views and these should be fully understood to optimize information obtained. From these radiographs, several parameters can be obtained to help evaluate patients before hip preservation surgery. These same radiographs can be helpful when considering revision hip arthroscopy and postoperative correction of deformity.

Anteroposterior (AP) pelvis radiograph is obtained routinely with patients positioned supine with the legs internally rotated by 15°. To allow optimal evaluation, the radiograph beam should be centered between the pubic symphysis and the anterior superior iliac spine.[2] AP pelvis radiographs are particularly useful for identification of the presence of osteoarthritis and measurement of joint space remaining to classify the degree of joint space loss. The Tönnis grade can be helpful to quantify the amount of joint space narrowing.[3] Patients with Tönnis grade 2 or more generally benefit less from hip preservation.[2] Several important radiographic parameters allow for detailed analysis of morphology on both the acetabular and femoral sides. These parameters should take into account the relative tilt of the pelvis and rotation by evaluating symmetry and bony relationships because this has a profound influence on acetabular version.[4]

Pincer-type FAI is appreciated on the AP radiograph by presence of acetabular retroversion, overcoverage, coxa profunda, protrusio acetabula, and increased anterior center-edge angle or lateral center-edge angle (LCEA).[5] Measurement of the lateral and anterior center-edge angle are helpful screening measures in most cases; however, there are abnormal acetabular morphologic variants that may not always be defined by these parameters. Measuring the LCEA and acetabular inclination angle (Tönnis angle) are measurements that can characterize acetabular morphology. Global overcoverage has been defined as an LCEA greater than 40° and Tönnis angle less than 0° (**Fig. 1**). Acetabular dysplasia can be defined by LCEA less than 20° and Tönnis angle greater than 10°. There are other radiographic findings that may be relevant, such as Shenton line, femoral version, and neck shaft angle.

Coxa profunda is now recognized as potentially a normal variant in many individuals.[6,7] Evaluation for acetabular dysplasia is crucial to successful patient selection.[8] When the center of the femoral head extends beyond the ilioischial line, acetabular protrusio may be present, representing global overcoverage of the femoral head.[9–11] Presuming a proper pelvic tilt on AP pelvic radiograph, a crossover sign denotes that the anterior wall of the acetabulum projects lateral to the posterior wall before converging at the lateral acetabular sourcil. Once a crossover sign is recognized, quantification can be achieved by measuring the retroversion index, which can be helpful in planning surgical correction.[10,12] A posterior wall sign indicates that the center of the femoral head projects lateral to the posterior wall, which is another sign of true

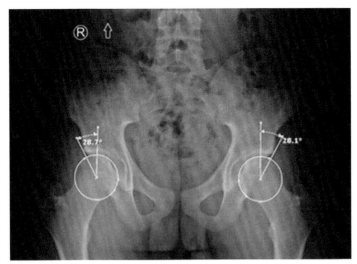

Fig. 1. AP pelvis radiograph demonstrating measurement of bi-LCEA in 16-year old male patient with FAI.

acetabular retroversion.[2] Although a posterior wall sign represents true acetabular retroversion, an isolated crossover sign may represent focal overcoverage by the anterior wall in pincer-type deformity.

Proximal femoral pathoanatomy is a 3D deformity that may be easily identified on plain radiographs in moderate to severe cases or, in subtle cases, may only be obvious on arthroscopic visualization. The alpha angle represents the most commonly used parameter (**Fig. 2**) with the alpha point representing where the deformity extends outside the best-fit circle.[13,14] In Notzli's original work,[15] symptomatic patients had

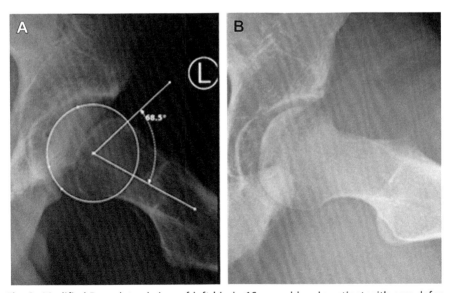

Fig. 2. Modified Dunn lateral view of left hip in 16-year-old male patient with cam deformity. (*A*) Alpha angle. (*B*) Modified Dunn lateral after cam resection.

an alpha angle averaging 74° compared with 42° in asymptomatic patients. Several other studies reported other ranges of normal.[9,15] Most orthopedic surgeons define a cam deformity as greater than 50° on any radiographic view. In some cases, the cam deformity is best appreciated on the AP view known as a pistol grip deformity.[16,17] The measurement of the alpha angle on the AP view is also known as the gamma angle. Further analysis can include quantitative complementary measurement of the patient's cam-type deformity and head neck offset.[2]

The authors recommend using a series of plain radiographs to visualize the proximal femoral anatomy in different positions. Each radiographic view needs to be scrutinized to identify an abnormal head neck offset. The authors' institutional preference is to use a combination of the AP pelvis, false-profile, and 90° Dunn lateral view; each of these can be used to measure cam morphology. In addition to characterizing the femoral head-neck junction, the false-profile view may be obtained to evaluate several parameters, including the morphology of the anterior inferior iliac spine.[18] Several variations of the lateral femoral view exist, including the 45° and 90° Dunn lateral, cross table lateral, and frog leg lateral. Other notable findings in symptomatic patients on plain radiographs may include impingement cysts and trough signs.

The importance of correlating radiographic findings to clinical symptoms cannot be overemphasized because a large portion of patients with FAI morphology may never become symptomatic. The literature suggests a high number of asymptomatic patients have radiographic measurements indicating FAI.[6,7]

COMPUTED TOMOGRAPHY

3D imaging allows for advanced characterization of the patient's bony morphology. Computed tomography (CT) can be profoundly helpful in surgical planning for FAI.[3,19] Advances in preoperative planning software and motion analysis technology based on advanced imaging represent a growing area of hip preservation surgery.[19,20] CT is helpful in further delineation of a bony pathologic state noted on plain radiographs, though routine use is controversial given the degree of radiation exposure.[21] This is a particularly important consideration in young patients who are being considered for FAI surgery.[3]

Acetabular version and pincer morphology can be appreciated at a high level on multiplanar or 3D CT reconstructions (**Fig. 3**).[22] When considering hip arthroscopy

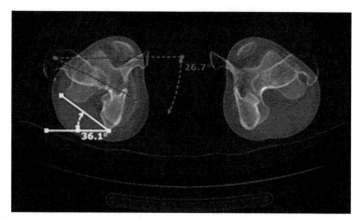

Fig. 3. CT measurement of femoral anteversion is performed by measuring the angle formed between the long axis of the femoral neck and a line parallel to the dorsal aspect of the femoral condyles on axial CT scan.

with femoral osteochondroplasty, the exact location of cam deformity can be determined with CT.[23] The CT scan can also obtain information about the proximal femoral version to characterize extra-articular deformity and impingement. 3D reconstructions can be rendered to allow for detailed assessment of areas of impingement, especially in the revision situation (**Fig. 4**).[24,25] Finally, when MRI is contraindicated, CT arthrography may represent an alternative to MRI for evaluation of labral and soft tissue disease, though MRI remains the gold standard for chondrolabral injury.

MAGNETIC RESONANCE IMAGING

MRI is a common diagnostic option to evaluate soft tissue hip injuries in patients undergoing workup for FAI. Imaging techniques include but are not limited to conventional noncontrast MRI, indirect magnetic resonance arthrography (MRA) and direct MRA. The latter techniques differ by route of contrast injection. Indirect MRA is intravenously injected; direct MRA is intra-articularly injected.[2] Routine imaging sequences include coronal fat-saturated T2 fast spin echo (FSE), coronal T1 FSE, sagittal proton density (PD) FSE, axial PD FSE, and FS axial oblique PD FSE, and radial PD FSE.[26,27] These multiplanar sequences and the excellent tissue contrast resolution of MRI or MRA demonstrates intra-articular soft tissue disease commonly seen with FAI, such as the acetabular labrum and articular cartilage. They also reveal extra-articular disease such as hip abductor tendinopathy or trochanteric inflammation associated with FAI.[28–32] In addition to soft tissue structures, MRI can be used to identify osseous pathomorphology, such as cam deformities, through radial or axial oblique slices, acetabular anteversion or retroversion, femoral head-neck offset, and femoral antetorsion. MRI is unique for the ability to demonstrate bone marrow edema or subchondral cysts before radiographic changes are seen.[26,27,33,34]

Evaluating for labral tears is an important diagnostic step in the work-up of FAI.[35] Several studies[36–38] have demonstrated that direct MRA increases sensitivity for assessing labral pathomorphology. Intra-articularly injected contrast distends the hip joint and promotes separation of the labrum from the hip capsule, thus enhancing visualization of labrum and associated disease.[39] The 2 prominent findings of labral tears are (1) contrast extending into the body of the labrum and (2) labral detachment from the acetabulum (**Fig. 5**). Although useful at categorizing different types of labral tears, Blankenbaker and colleagues[40] found poor correlation between the original

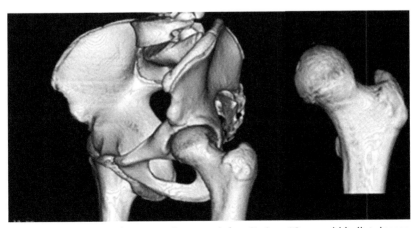

Fig. 4. 3D reconstructions demonstrating cam deformity in a 16-year-old ballet dancer.

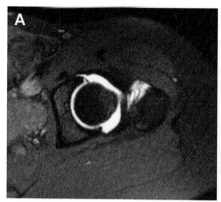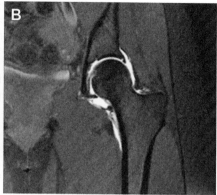

Fig. 5. Axial (*A*) and coronal (*B*) MRI arthrogram images demonstrating an anterolateral labral tear of the left hip.

classification by Czerny and colleagues[41] and the Lage arthroscopic classification system.[42] The latter is performed intra-operatively and segregates labral tears into radial flap tears, radial fibrillated tears, longitudinal peripheral tears, or unstable tears.[29,40,42] To address this, Blankenbaker and colleagues[40] proposed a descriptive system in which labral tears were divided into frayed, flap, peripheral longitudinal, and unstable. Location and extent of tears in this study[40] were determined using the clock-face localization system. In their study of 65 hip MRAs, Blankenbaker and colleagues[40] found 54% of labral tears isolated between the anterosuperior 12 to 3 o'clock position, with an additional 40% of tears involving this region but extending outside of it.[40]

Although MRA has shown to have high sensitivity for identifying labral disease, normal morphologic variants exist that can potentially obscure the workup of hip pain and FAI.[43] In a study of 200 asymptomatic subjects, Lecouvet and colleagues[43] found heterogeneity in both labral shape (66% triangular, 11% round, 9% flat) and signal intensity. Paralabral sulci and acetabular clefts have also been described as normal variants and are not to be confused with labral detachments or tears.[44] The incidence of sublabral sulci is roughly 20%.[45,46] They can be distinguished from tears by the relatively decreased depth, less signal intensity, and an absence of paralabral cysts or cartilage damage.[27,39,45,46] Just as important is that abnormal findings can be present in asymptomatic individuals. In a recent study of 45 asymptomatic hips, Register and colleagues[1] identified labral tears in 69%, chondral defects in 24%, and paralabral cysts in 13%.[1] Further, the incidence of labral tears in the asymptomatic population has been reported as high as 83% in 1 cohort.[47] Thus, when assessing labral morphology, correlation between clinical and imaging findings must be stressed.

Cartilage damage is also frequent in FAI and, until recently, MRI had less diagnostic usefulness for evaluating chondral lesions. Traditional MRI of the hip articular cartilage is impeded by limited cartilage thickness, its complex 3D geometry, and the close apposition between the femoral head and acetabular cartilage layers.[48] In comparison to the greater than 90% sensitivity of MRA in detecting labral tears, Anderson and colleagues[49] report a 22% sensitivity for MRA to detect cartilage delamination. Pfirrman and colleagues[30] report a similarly low sensitivity (26%) when using hyperintense fluid signal beneath the cartilage to define delamination but a higher sensitivity (63%, with 90% specificity) when defining delamination by hypointense areas in the acetabular cartilage on coronal intermediate weighted fat-saturated images. Despite improvements in imaging protocol and technique, the ability of conventional MRI or MRA to detect cartilage pathomorphology in the hip remains limited to identifying gross lesions.[27]

ROLE OF IMAGING IN PREOPERATIVE PLANNING

Following an appropriate and thorough history and physical examination, diagnostic imaging plays an important role in determining the correct diagnosis for the young patient with hip pain.[50] Recognition and correlation of physical examination findings with bony and soft tissue abnormalities identified on diagnostic imaging allows the surgeon to appreciate the unique fingerprint of disease in each patient. Preoperatively identifying the individualized pathologic condition helps to devise a preoperative plan for adequate treatment. This section outlines the standard preoperative imaging assessment implemented by the senior author (SJN).

The imaging assessment of every patient that presents with hip or groin pain begins with plain radiographs. Standardized radiographs are mandatory and care is taken to ensure correct film-focus distance and proper centering of the radiograph beam to prevent alteration of the osseous anatomy and thus false impressions.[3,51]

The senior author's preferred initial radiographs include a true AP radiograph of the pelvis and 2 lateral views of the affected hip. The lateral views include a 90° Dunn lateral and a false-profile lateral. The AP of the pelvis is used to evaluate the focal and global overcoverage of the hip joint, as well as the acetabular rim morphology.[51] In addition, the AP pelvis and false-profile views can be used to determine if there are signs of hip dysplasia. The false-profile view is valuable to gain information regarding the magnitude of anterior acetabular coverage in addition to denoting any signs of potential subspine impingement.[52,53] The assessment of the proximal femur is conducted on the AP pelvis (assessing the most lateral aspect of any cam morphology) and on the 2 lateral views (assessing increasingly more anterior aspects of any cam morphology).[15] The false-profile view has been most strongly correlated to characterization of cam deformity at the 2 o'clock and 3 o'clock positions on CT scan.[18] The false-profile view combined with AP pelvis and 90 Dunn lateral view of the hip comprise a good screening radiographic series for patients presenting with symptoms of FAI. In addition to calculating an alpha angle, the head-neck offset and femoral neck-shaft angle can calculated.[3]

In young, active patients with symptomatic FAI determined by initial radiographs, the authors use advanced imaging modalities to preoperatively plan the osseous resection and concomitant soft tissue procedures. We currently use CT scanning of the hip to obtain a 3D representation of the osseous morphology of the proximal femur and acetabulum independent of patient positioning. A benefit of CT compared with plain radiographs is the ability to more accurately measure the degree of focal or global acetabular coverage.[4,54] On the femoral-side, we use CT to further characterize the 3D morphology of the cam deformity. CT has been shown to improve surgeons' intraobserver and interobserver reliability of measurable FAI parameters compared with plain radiographs.[22,55] MRI is also routinely used in preoperative planning. With proper sequencing techniques, noncontrast MRI is comparable to MRA and without the additional invasiveness and cost.[56] At the authors' institution, MRA is the preferred method to evaluate for the intra-articular soft tissue structures of the hip. This modality is used to identify labral tears, chondral delamination and degeneration, capsular deficiency (**Fig. 6**), and other soft tissue abnormalities that can be addressed at the time of surgery.[57]

Finally, in symptomatic patients with either multiple possible sources of pain or in patients where the diagnosis is unclear, image-guided injections can be used for

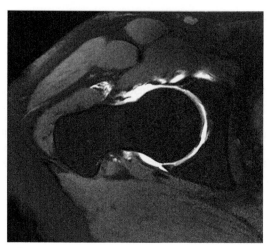

Fig. 6. Axial MRI arthrogram in a 36-year-old female patient with microinstability and persistent pain after a previous hip arthroscopy. MRI demonstrates contrast extravasation and a persistent capsular defect.

both diagnostic and therapeutic purposes. Compared with blind injections, image-guided injections are safer, more accurate, and result in better clinical outcomes.[58] Relief of pain after an intra-articular injection is 90% reliable as an indicator for intra-articular hip pathologic condition and may predict improved outcomes following surgery.[59,60] The authors' preferred injection procedure is to perform an examination of the patient before the injection, and repeat the examination after the injection to quantify the extent of relief.

IMAGING PARAMETERS OF SUCCESSFUL FEMOROACETABULAR IMPINGEMENT CORRECTION

Incomplete resection of underlying FAI deformity is a major reason for residual hip pain following surgery and a leading cause of revision hip arthroscopy.[24,25,61–64] Over-resection of offending osseous disease may lead to iatrogenic instability and poor outcomes.[61,65,66] In addition to careful attention to preoperative imaging, recent research has suggested that systematic implementation of intraoperative fluoroscopy can assist in providing adequate acetabular and femoral decompression and avoid the most common cause of revision hip arthroscopy.[23,67–69]

When addressing the acetabular correction of pincer-type FAI, recent research has demonstrated that small resections on the order of 5 to 10 mm make large changes in center-edge angle measurements.[67,68,70] Kling and colleagues[67] concluded that a 1 mm resection will decrease the LCEA by 1° and the anterior center-edge angle by 2°. This formula may be used intra-operatively to balance the line between adequate rim resection and iatrogenic instability. The authors also use the anterior margin ratio to quantify the amount of acetabular overcoverage on intra-operative fluoroscopy to guide the amount of rim resection. Similarly, intraoperative techniques exist to ensure adequate femoral-sided decompression. Ross and colleagues[23] implemented an accurate and reproducible approach to obtain 6 fluoroscopic views to confirm complete cam resection. Each of the 6 intraoperative fluoroscopic views corresponds to a standardized right hip clock-face position, which is the most common nomenclature for discussing FAI position.[21,71,72] The femoral head-neck region covered by the

6 radiographic views (11:45–2:45) has been documented as the region most commonly associated with cam pathologic condition.[33,57,64,73] In similar fashion to acetabular-sided decompression, intraoperative use of fluoroscopy on the femoral side aids in balancing the fine line between under-resection, leading to residual pain, and over-resection, leading to femoral neck fracture.[24,25,61–64,74,75]

FUTURE DIRECTIONS

Cartilage disease may be predictive of poorer outcomes after hip preservation surgery. Despite the limitations of conventional MRI, recent advances in biochemical imaging techniques have shown promise for detecting cartilage disease earlier and on a microscopic level.[76–79] These techniques include quantitative T2 and T2* relaxation mapping to assess cartilage water content and collagen organization,[77,80] as well as T1rho (T1ρ)[78] and delayed gadolinium-enhanced MRI of cartilage (dGEMRIC)[81] techniques to evaluate proteoglycan content. dGEMRIC studies require injection of a negatively charged gadolinium contrast agent, which distributes according to the negative charge of extracellular glycosaminoglycans. Areas of diseased cartilage with lower proteoglycan content (and higher water content) will, therefore, have higher amounts of contrast and shorter $T1_{Gd}$ relaxation time (**Fig. 7**).[82] dGEMRIC is capable of detecting cartilage damage in patients with FAI,[81,83] as well as in asymptomatic patients with cam deformities.[84] When injected intra-articularly, it can combine the advantages of dGEMRIC for cartilage assessment with arthrography for labral evaluation.[85]

T1ρ imaging techniques also assess the relative glycosaminoglycan of hyaline cartilage but do not require the contrast injection. Despite a paucity in the literature on this topic, available studies suggest that T1ρ can detect articular cartilage abnormalities in patients with FAI, as well as in asymptomatic patients with cam deformities.[78,86,87] Although promising, preliminary imaging studies require replication and standardization to increase the applicability of these developing techniques.[79]

Patient-specific 3D models of the hip using commercially available 3D CT rendering software have been developed and may allow clinicians to perform dynamic analysis of the hip. This analysis has been used to identify mechanical impingement in a patient's range of motion, including sports-specific positions, which may then be used

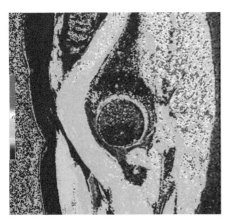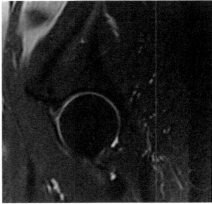

Fig. 7. dGEMRIC (*left*) and sagittal T2 weighted MRI images (*right*) demonstrating well-preserved cartilage in a 36-year-old patient being considered for revision hip arthroscopy.

In a preoperative plan to plan the bony resection. Many investigators suggest this type of individualized plan of care is the way of the future because it may increase precision and decrease radiation.

SUMMARY

Hip arthroscopy continues to experience incredible growth and advances in imaging have progressed concomitantly. Plain radiographs play a key role in initial management of patients presenting with hip pain when FAI is suspected. 3D imaging with CT and MRI allows for advanced characterization of the patient's bony morphology and soft tissue injury. Incomplete resection of underlying FAI deformity is a major reason for residual hip pain following surgery and a leading cause of revision hip arthroscopy. A comprehensive approach to preoperative and intraoperative assessment of FAI treatment portends the best outcome.

REFERENCES

1. Register B, Pennock AT, Ho CP, et al. Prevalence of abnormal hip findings in asymptomatic participants: a prospective, blinded study. Am J Sports Med 2012;40:2720–4.
2. Nepple JJ, Prather H, Trousdale RT, et al. Diagnostic imaging of femoroacetabular impingement. J Am Acad Orthop Surg 2013;21(Suppl 1):S20–6.
3. Clohisy JC, Carlisle JC, Beaulé PE, et al. A systematic approach to the plain radiographic evaluation of the young adult hip. J Bone Joint Surg Am 2008;90: 47–66.
4. Zaltz I, Kelly BT, Hetsroni I, et al. The crossover sign overestimates acetabular retroversion. Clin Orthop Relat Res 2013;471:2463–70.
5. Bedi A, Kelly BT. Femoroacetabular impingement. J Bone Joint Surg Am 2013;95: 82–92.
6. Frank JM, Harris JD, Erickson BJ, et al. Prevalence of femoroacetabular impingement imaging findings in asymptomatic volunteers: a systematic review. Arthroscopy 2015;31:1199–204.
7. Diesel CV, Ribeiro TA, Coussirat C, et al. Coxa profunda in the diagnosis of pincer-type femoroacetabular impingement and its prevalence in asymptomatic subjects. Bone Joint J 2015;97-B:478–83.
8. Harris JD, Gerrie BJ, Varner KE, et al. Radiographic Prevalence of Dysplasia, Cam, and Pincer Deformities in Elite Ballet. Am J Sports Med 2016;44(1):20–7.
9. Ganz R, Parvizi J, Beck M, et al. Femoroacetabular impingement: a cause for osteoarthritis of the hip. Clin Orthop Relat Res 2003;(417):112–20.
10. Fadul DA, Carrino JA. Imaging of femoroacetabular impingement. J Bone Joint Surg Am 2009;91(Suppl 1):138–43.
11. Byrd JWT, Jones KS. Arthroscopic management of femoroacetabular impingement: minimum 2-year follow-up. Arthroscopy 2011;27:1379–88.
12. Gebhart JJ, Streit JJ, Bedi A, et al. Correlation of pelvic incidence with cam and pincer lesions. Am J Sports Med 2014;42:2649–53.
13. Ng VY, Ellis TJ. Cam morphology in the human hip. Orthopedics 2012;35:320–7.
14. Laborie LB, Lehmann TG, Engesæter IØ, et al. The alpha angle in cam-type femoroacetabular impingement: new reference intervals based on 2038 healthy young adults. Bone Joint J 2014;96-B:449–54.
15. Nötzli HP, Wyss TF, Stoecklin CH, et al. The contour of the femoral head-neck junction as a predictor for the risk of anterior impingement. J Bone Joint Surg Br 2002;84:556–60.

16. Ilizaliturri VM, Orozco-Rodriguez L, Acosta-Rodríguez E, et al. Arthroscopic treatment of cam-type femoroacetabular impingement: preliminary report at 2 years minimum follow-up. J Arthroplasty 2008;23:226–34.

17. Mellado JM, Radi N. Cam-type deformities: Concepts, criteria, and multidetector CT features. Radiologia 2015;57:213–24.

18. Hellman MD, Mascarenhas R, Gupta A, et al. The false-profile view may be used to identify cam morphology. Arthroscopy 2015;31:1728–32.

19. Heyworth BE, Dolan MM, Nguyen JT, et al. Preoperative three-dimensional CT predicts intraoperative findings in hip arthroscopy. Clin Orthop Relat Res 2012; 470:1950–7.

20. Tannenbaum EP, Ross JR, Bedi A. Pros, cons, and future possibilities for use of computer navigation in hip arthroscopy. Sports Med Arthrosc 2014;22:e33–41.

21. Nepple JJ, Martel JM, Kim YJ, et al. Do plain radiographs correlate with CT for imaging of cam-type femoroacetabular impingement? Clin Orthop Relat Res 2012;470:3313–20.

22. Cadet ER, Babatunde OM, Gorroochurn P, et al. Inter- and intra-observer agreement of femoroacetabular impingement (FAI) parameters comparing plain radiographs and advanced, 3D computed tomographic (CT)-generated hip models in a surgical patient cohort. Knee Surg Sports Traumatol Arthrosc 2014. http://dx.doi.org/10.1007/s00167-014-3315-8.

23. Ross JR, Bedi A, Stone RM, et al. Intraoperative fluoroscopic imaging to treat cam deformities: correlation with 3-dimensional computed tomography. Am J Sports Med 2014;42:1370–6.

24. Larson CM, Giveans MR, Samuelson KM, et al. Arthroscopic Hip Revision Surgery for Residual Femoroacetabular Impingement (FAI): Surgical Outcomes Compared With a Matched Cohort After Primary Arthroscopic FAI Correction. Am J Sports Med 2014;42:1785–90.

25. Philippon MJ, Schenker ML, Briggs KK, et al. Revision hip arthroscopy. Am J Sports Med 2007;35:1918–21.

26. Bredella MA, Ulbrich EJ, Stoller DW, et al. Femoroacetabular impingement. Magn Reson Imaging Clin N Am 2013;21:45–64.

27. Riley GM, McWalter EJ, Stevens KJ, et al. MRI of the hip for the evaluation of femoroacetabular impingement; past, present, and future. J Magn Reson Imaging 2015;41:558–72.

28. Leunig M, Podeszwa D, Beck M, et al. Magnetic resonance arthrography of labral disorders in hips with dysplasia and impingement. Clin Orthop Relat Res 2004;(418):74–80.

29. Freedman BA, Potter BK, Dinauer PA, et al. Prognostic value of magnetic resonance arthrography for Czerny stage II and III acetabular labral tears. Arthroscopy 2006;22:742–7.

30. Pfirrmann CWA, Duc SR, Zanetti M, et al. MR arthrography of acetabular cartilage delamination in femoroacetabular cam impingement. Radiology 2008;249:236–41.

31. Klontzas ME, Karantanas AH. Greater trochanter pain syndrome: a descriptive MR imaging study. Eur J Radiol 2014;83:1850–5.

32. Cvitanic O, Henzie G, Skezas N, et al. MRI diagnosis of tears of the hip abductor tendons (gluteus medius and gluteus minimus). AJR Am J Roentgenol 2004;182:137–43.

33. Rakhra KS, Sheikh AM, Allen D, et al. Comparison of MRI alpha angle measurement planes in femoroacetabular impingement. Clin Orthop Relat Res 2009;467:660–5.

34. Dimmick S, Stevens KJ, Brazier D, et al. Femoroacetabular impingement. Radiol Clin North Am 2013;51:337–52.

35. Meermans G, Konan S, Haddad FS, et al. Prevalence of acetabular cartilage lesions and labral tears in femoroacetabular impingement. Acta Orthop Belg 2010;76:181–8.

36. Smith TO, Simpson M, Ejindu V, et al. The diagnostic test accuracy of magnetic resonance imaging, magnetic resonance arthrography and computer tomography in the detection of chondral lesions of the hip. Eur J Orthop Surg Traumatol 2013;23:335–44.

37. Toomayan GA, Holman WR, Major NM, et al. Sensitivity of MR arthrography in the evaluation of acetabular labral tears. AJR Am J Roentgenol 2006;186:449–53.

38. Tian C-Y, Wang J-Q, Zheng Z-Z, et al. 3.0 T conventional hip MR and hip MR arthrography for the acetabular labral tears confirmed by arthroscopy. Eur J Radiol 2014;83:1822–7.

39. Thomas JD, Li Z, Agur AM, et al. Imaging of the acetabular labrum. Semin Musculoskelet Radiol 2013;17:248–57.

40. Blankenbaker DG, De Smet AA, Keene JS, et al. Classification and localization of acetabular labral tears. Skeletal Radiol 2007;36:391–7.

41. Czerny C, Hofmann S, Neuhold A, et al. Lesions of the acetabular labrum: accuracy of MR imaging and MR arthrography in detection and staging. Radiology 1996;200:225–30.

42. Lage LA, Patel JV, Villar RN. The acetabular labral tear: an arthroscopic classification. Arthroscopy 1996;12:269–72.

43. Lecouvet FE, Vande Berg BC, Malghem J, et al. MR imaging of the acetabular labrum: variations in 200 asymptomatic hips. AJR Am J Roentgenol 1996;167:1025–8.

44. DuBois DF, Omar IM. MR imaging of the hip: normal anatomic variants and imaging pitfalls. Magn Reson Imaging Clin N Am 2010;18:663–74.

45. Dinauer PA, Murphy KP, Carroll JF. Sublabral sulcus at the posteroinferior acetabulum: a potential pitfall in MR arthrography diagnosis of acetabular labral tears. AJR Am J Roentgenol 2004;183:1745–53.

46. Studler U, Kalberer F, Leunig M, et al. MR arthrography of the hip: differentiation between an anterior sublabral recess as a normal variant and a labral tear. Radiology 2008;249:947–54.

47. Schmitz MR, Campbell SE, Fajardo RS, et al. Identification of acetabular labral pathological changes in asymptomatic volunteers using optimized, noncontrast 1.5-T magnetic resonance imaging. Am J Sports Med 2012;40:1337–41.

48. Link TM, Schwaiger BJ, Zhang AL. Regional Articular Cartilage Abnormalities of the Hip. Am J Roentgenol 2015;205:502–12.

49. Anderson LA, Peters CL, Park BB, et al. Acetabular cartilage delamination in femoroacetabular impingement. Risk factors and magnetic resonance imaging diagnosis. J Bone Joint Surg Am 2009;91:305–13.

50. Skendzel JG, Weber AE, Ross JR, et al. The approach to the evaluation and surgical treatment of mechanical hip pain in the young patient: AAOS exhibit selection. J Bone Joint Surg Am 2013;95:e133.

51. Tannast M, Siebenrock KA, Anderson SE. Femoroacetabular impingement: radiographic diagnosis—what the radiologist should know. Am J Roentgenol 2007;188:1540–52.

52. Garbuz DS, Masri BA, Haddad F, et al. Clinical and radiographic assessment of the young adult with symptomatic hip dysplasia. Clin Orthop Relat Res 2004;(418):18–22.

53. Larson CM, Kelly BT, Stone RM. Making a case for anterior inferior iliac spine/subspine hip impingement: three representative case reports and proposed concept. Arthroscopy 2011;27:1732–7.

54. Larson CM, Moreau-Gaudry A, Kelly BT, et al. Are normal hips being labeled as pathologic? A CT-based method for defining normal acetabular coverage. Clin Orthop Relat Res 2015;473:1247–54.

55. Milone MT, Bedi A, Poultsides L, et al. Novel CT-based three-dimensional software improves the characterization of cam morphology. Clin Orthop Relat Res 2013;471:2484–91.

56. Mintz DN, Hooper T, Connell D, et al. Magnetic resonance imaging of the hip: detection of labral and chondral abnormalities using noncontrast imaging. Arthroscopy 2005;21:385–93.

57. Pfirrmann CWA, Mengiardi B, Dora C, et al. Cam and pincer femoroacetabular impingement: characteristic MR arthrographic findings in 50 patients. Radiology 2006;240:778–85.

58. Epis O, Bruschi E. Interventional ultrasound: a critical overview on ultrasound-guided injections and biopsies. Clin Exp Rheumatol 2014;32:S78–84.

59. Byrd JWT, Jones KS. Diagnostic accuracy of clinical assessment, magnetic resonance imaging, magnetic resonance arthrography, and intra-articular injection in hip arthroscopy patients. Am J Sports Med 2004;32:1668–74.

60. Ayeni OR, Farrokhyar F, Crouch S, et al. Pre-operative intra-articular hip injection as a predictor of short-term outcome following arthroscopic management of femoroacetabular impingement. Knee Surg Sports Traumatol Arthrosc 2014;22: 801–5.

61. Bogunovic L, Gottlieb M, Pashos G, et al. Why do hip arthroscopy procedures fail? Clin Orthop Relat Res 2013;471:2523–9.

62. Clohisy JC, Nepple JJ, Larson CM, et al. Persistent structural disease is the most common cause of repeat hip preservation surgery. Clin Orthop Relat Res 2013; 471:3788–94.

63. Heyworth BE, Shindle MK, Voos JE, et al. Radiologic and intraoperative findings in revision hip arthroscopy. Arthroscopy 2007;23:1295–302.

64. Ross JR, Larson CM, Adeoye O, et al. Residual deformity is the most common reason for revision hip arthroscopy: a three-dimensional CT study. Clin Orthop Relat Res 2015;473:1388–95.

65. Benali Y, Katthagen BD. Hip subluxation as a complication of arthroscopic debridement. Arthroscopy 2009;25:405–7.

66. Matsuda DK. Acute iatrogenic dislocation following hip impingement arthroscopic surgery. Arthroscopy 2009;25:400–4.

67. Kling S, Karns MR, Gebhart J, et al. The effect of acetabular rim recession on anterior acetabular coverage: a cadaveric study using the false-profile radiograph. Am J Sports Med 2015;43:957–64.

68. Philippon MJ, Wolff AB, Briggs KK, et al. Acetabular rim reduction for the treatment of femoroacetabular impingement correlates with preoperative and postoperative center-edge angle. Arthroscopy 2010;26:757–61.

69. Matsuda DK. Fluoroscopic templating technique for precision arthroscopic rim trimming. Arthroscopy 2009;25:1175–82.

70. Colvin AC, Koehler SM, Bird J. Can the change in center-edge angle during pincer trimming be reliably predicted? Clin Orthop Relat Res 2011;469:1071–4.

71. Philippon MJ, Stubbs AJ, Schenker ML, et al. Arthroscopic management of femoroacetabular impingement osteoplasty technique and literature review. Am J Sports Med 2007;35:1571–80.

72. Illzaliturri VM, Byrd JW, Sampson TG, et al. A geographic zone method to describe intra-articular pathology in hip arthroscopy: cadaveric study and preliminary report. Arthroscopy 2008;24:534–9.

73. Ito K, Minka MA, Leunig M, et al. Femoroacetabular impingement and the cam-effect. A MRI-based quantitative anatomical study of the femoral head-neck offset. J Bone Joint Surg Br 2001;83:171–6.

74. Sampson TG. Complications of hip arthroscopy. Clin Sports Med 2001;20:831–5.

75. Harris JD, McCormick FM, Abrams GD, et al. Complications and reoperations during and after hip arthroscopy: a systematic review of 92 studies and more than 6,000 patients. Arthroscopy 2013;29:589–95.

76. Lattanzi R, Petchprapa C, Glaser C, et al. A new method to analyze dGEMRIC measurements in femoroacetabular impingement: preliminary validation against arthroscopic findings. Osteoarthritis Cartilage 2012;20:1127–33.

77. Watanabe A, Boesch C, Siebenrock K, et al. T2 mapping of hip articular cartilage in healthy volunteers at 3T: a study of topographic variation. J Magn Reson Imaging 2007;26:165–71.

78. Rakhra KS, Lattanzio P-J, Cárdenas-Blanco A, et al. Can T1-rho MRI detect acetabular cartilage degeneration in femoroacetabular impingement?: a pilot study. J Bone Joint Surg Br 2012;94:1187–92.

79. Bittersohl B, Hosalkar HS, Hesper T, et al. Advanced imaging in femoroacetabular impingement: current state and future prospects. Front Surg 2015;2:34.

80. Bittersohl B, Hosalkar HS, Hughes T, et al. Feasibility of T2* mapping for the evaluation of hip joint cartilage at 1.5T using a three-dimensional (3D), gradient-echo (GRE) sequence: A prospective study. Magn Reson Med 2009;62:896–901.

81. Bittersohl B, Steppacher S, Haamberg T, et al. Cartilage damage in femoroacetabular impingement (FAI): preliminary results on comparison of standard diagnostic vs delayed gadolinium-enhanced magnetic resonance imaging of cartilage (dGEMRIC). Osteoarthritis Cartilage 2009;17:1297–306.

82. Bashir A, Gray ML, Boutin RD, et al. Glycosaminoglycan in articular cartilage: in vivo assessment with delayed Gd(DTPA)(2-)-enhanced MR imaging. Radiology 1997;205:551–8.

83. Mamisch TC, Kain MS, Bittersohl B, et al. Delayed gadolinium-enhanced magnetic resonance imaging of cartilage (dGEMRIC) in Femoacetabular impingement. J Orthop Res 2011;29:1305–11.

84. Pollard TCB, McNally EG, Wilson DC, et al. Localized cartilage assessment with three-dimensional dGEMRIC in asymptomatic hips with normal morphology and cam deformity. J Bone Joint Surg Am 2010;92:2557–69.

85. Zilkens C, Miese F, Kim YJ, et al. Direct comparison of intra-articular versus intravenous delayed gadolinium-enhanced MRI of hip joint cartilage. J Magn Reson Imaging 2014;39:94–102.

86. Subburaj K, Valentinitsch A, Dillon AB, et al. Regional variations in MR relaxation of hip joint cartilage in subjects with and without femoralacetabular impingement. Magn Reson Imaging 2013;31:1129–36.

87. Anwander H, Melkus G, Rakhra KS, et al. T1ρ MRI detects cartilage damage in asymptomatic individuals with a cam deformity. J Orthop Res 2015. http://dx.doi.org/10.1002/jor.23101.

Management of the Acetabular Labrum

Andrew B. Wolff, MD[a],*, Jamie Grossman, MD[b]

KEYWORDS

- Acetabular labrum • Labral reconstruction • Labral repair • Labral debridement
- Hip preservation

KEY POINTS

- The acetabular labrum is a biomechanically important structure that stabilizes the hip and protects the articular cartilage.
- The labrum has free nerve fibers and can be a pain generator.
- Painless restoration of normal hip biomechanics should be the goal of clinical correction of labral dysfunction through labral debridement, labral repair, or labral reconstruction.
- Labral debridement, repair, and reconstruction can be viable treatment options in the correct clinical setting.

INTRODUCTION

A normal-functioning acetabular labrum can be an important component of a stable, long-lasting, and well-functioning hip joint. A compromised labrum can be the source of significant disability and pain. Painless restoration of normal hip biomechanics should be the goal of arthroscopic treatment of labral dysfunction through labral debridement, repair, or reconstruction.

Biomechanically, multiple in vivo studies have demonstrated the function of the labrum. Ferguson and colleagues[1,2] demonstrated that the labrum distributes joint forces, stabilizes the hip, and acts as a seal to promote lubrication and preserve cartilage, and with its removal, the articular cartilage layers compress 40% more quickly. Other investigators have shown that the labrum contributes to hip stability by increasing acetabular surface area, volume, and stiffness, and by creating a negative intra-articular pressure that results in resistance to displacement.[3] The hip fluid seal provided by the labrum maintains pressure within the joint to protect the cartilage

Disclosure Statement: Dr A.B. Wolff is a Consultant for Stryker. There is no commercial bias in the material of this article.
[a] Department of Orthopedic Surgery, Washington Orthopaedics and Sports Medicine, 2021 K Street Northwest, Suite 516, Washington, DC 20006, USA; [b] Department of Orthopaedic Surgery, Lenox Hill Hospital, 210 East 64th Street, New York, NY 10065, USA
* Corresponding author.
E-mail address: andywolffmd@gmail.com

matrix from as much as 90% of the load and decreases friction between the femoral head and acetabulum.[4,5]

To restore these labral functions, 3 surgical options exist: debridement, repair, and reconstruction. Historically, debridement was the only option. In 2006, Espinosa and colleagues[6] demonstrated superior results among patients in whom the labrum was refixed to the acetabular rim after open surgical dislocation for correction of femoroacetabular impingement (FAI). In this study, only 28% of the resection group had excellent results, whereas 80% of the labral reattachment group had excellent results. This work, in concert with improved arthroscopic instrumentation and techniques, led to an attempt to preserve the labrum and restore its anatomy and function to approximate that of a "normal" hip. In 2009, Larson[7] reported superior outcomes among his patients who underwent arthroscopic refixation of the labrum versus debridement. Of the patients in the refixation group, 89% had good to excellent results compared with only 66% of patients who underwent debridement. These results have continued to be superior at midterm follow-up (92% vs 68%).[8] Several studies have supported these findings and demonstrated significantly better clinical outcomes with repair when compared with resection or debridement.[8,9]

Understanding that patients generally fare better with a repair and that the hip has improved mechanical properties with a functioning labrum led to the development of labral reconstruction techniques as an option for patients with labral tissue that was missing or damaged beyond repair. Although labral reconstruction had been reported in a case series of 5 surgical dislocations,[10] Philippon and colleagues[11] were the first to describe their promising early results in a large series with arthroscopic labral reconstruction in patients without osteoarthritis.[12] More recently, White and colleagues[13] showed excellent 2-year results in a series of 152 consecutive hips that underwent arthroscopic labral reconstruction. Domb and colleagues[14] found significantly better results in patients undergoing arthroscopic labral reconstruction compared to those undergoing labral resection for labra damaged beyond repair as measured by Non-arthritic Hip Score (NAHS) and hip outcome score (HOS)-activities of daily living (ADL) scores. Taking it a step farther, Matsuda and Burchette[15] compared their results with arthroscopic labral reconstruction with refixation in a matched cohort study and found that NAHS scores were significantly higher in the reconstruction group at 2-year follow-up. Similarly, Wolff and colleagues[16] recently reported on 1-year follow-up in a consecutive series of 107 patients, that the 46 who underwent circumferential labral reconstruction had an improvement across all outcome measures statistically indistinguishable from the patients who underwent labral repair despite being significantly older with more severe labral damage (or deficiency). Furthermore, in the reconstruction group, 35% were revisions compared with 3% of the repair group[16] (**Table 1**).

DEBRIDEMENT, REPAIR, RECONSTRUCTION: DOES IT MATTER?

Although there is a substantial and growing body of evidence that suggests both labral repair and reconstruction (probably more so than debridement) can help patients with hip pain, these treatments are not often performed in isolation. Increasing numbers of labral repairs among reporting investigators have historically paralleled not only advances in our understanding and ability to treat other conditions of the hip often performed concomitantly (ie, correction of FAI), but also a refinement of techniques, of patient selection, and a more thorough understanding of rehabilitation. Thus, some portion of the historically inferior results with labral debridement is likely attributable to the learning curves of both individual hip surgeons and the community of hip concept.

Table 1
Published open and arthroscopic labral reconstruction outcomes

Study	Open vs Arthroscopic/Graft	n	Sex	Age	Follow-up	Convert to THA	Preoperative Outcome	Postoperative Outcome
Sierra and Trousdale	Open/ligamentum teres capitis autograft	5	3 M, 2 F	33 (19–50) y	10 (5–20) mo	1 (20%)	• 3 "severe pain" • 2 "moderately severe pain" • UCLA: 5 (2–6)	• 3 "no pain" • 1 "moderate pain" • 1 "same pain as preoperatively" • UCLA: 8 (6–10)
Walker et al	Open/ligamentum teres capitis autograft or fascia lata autograft	20	5 M, 14 F	29 (16–50) y	26 (12–56) mo	3 (15%)	Not reported	• UCLA: 8.5 (5–10)
White et al	Arthroscopic/iliotibial band allograft	152	64 M, 78 F	39 (16–58) y	28 (24–39) mo	13 (10%)	• MHHS: 54 • LEFS: 41 • VAS rest: 5 • VAS ADLs: 6 • VAS sport: 8	• MHHS: 88 • LEFS: 68 • VAS rest: 2 • VAS ADLs: 2 • VAS sport: 3 • Satisfaction: 9/10
Philippon et al	Arthroscopic/iliotibial band autograft	47	32 M, 15 F	37 (18–55) y	18 (12–32) mo	4 (9%)	• MHHS: 62	• MHHS: 85 • Satisfaction: 8/10
Geyer et al	Arthroscopic/iliotibial band autograft	76	42 M, 33 F	39 (18–64) y	49 (36–70) mo	18 (24%) + 1 (1%) resurface	• MHHS: 59 • HOS-ADL: 69 • HOS-Sport: 41 • SF-12 physical: 42 • SF-12 mental: 55	• MHHS: 83 • HOS-ADL: 81 • HOS-Sport: 67 • SF-12 physical: 50 • SF-12 mental: 53 • Satisfaction: 8/10

(continued on next page)

Table 1
(continued)

Study	Open vs Arthroscopic/Graft	n	Sex	Age	Follow-up	Convert to THA	Preoperative Outcome	Postoperative Outcome
Boykin et al	Arthroscopic/iliotibial band autograft	21	19 M, 0 F	28 (19–41) y	41 (20–74) mo	2 (10%)	• MHHS: 67 • HOS-ADL: 77 • HOS-Sport: 56 • SF-12 physical: 44 • SF-12 mental: 49	• MHHS: 84 • HOS-ADL: 85 • HOS-Sport: 77 • SF-12 physical: 51 • SF-12 mental: 54 • Satisfaction: 8/10 • Returned to play: 18 (86%)
Matsuda and Burchette	Arthroscopic/gracilis autograft	8	7 M, 1 F	35 (18–58) y	30 (24–37) mo	0 (0%)	• NAHS: 42	• NAHS: 92 • Satisfaction: 7 "high," 1 "moderate"
Domb et al	Arthroscopic/gracilis tendon autograft	11	7 M, 4 F	33 (18–45) y	26 (24–32) mo	0 (0%)	• NAHS: 53 • HOS-ADL: 59 • HOS-Sport: 39 • MHHS: 55 • VAS: 7	• NAHS: 78 • HOS-ADL: 80 • HOS-Sport: 60 • MHHS: 82 • VAS: 3 • Satisfaction: 8/10

Abbreviations: ADLs, activities of daily living; HOS-ADL, hip outcome score-activities of daily living; HOS-Sport, hip outcome score-sports-specific subscale; NAHS, nonarthritic hip score; MHHS, modified Harris hip score; SF-12 mental, short form-12 mental component; SF-12 physical, short form-12 physical component; VAS, visual analog scale for pain.

Data are expressed as count (%) or mean (range).

From White BJ, Herzog MM. Labral reconstruction: when to perform and how. Front Surg 2015;2:27.

surgeons at large. Furthermore, as evidenced by most patients doing well with labral debridement and from studies such as that of Register and colleagues[17] finding labral tears in 69% of asymptomatic individuals on MRI, we know that there are many people who can tolerate an imperfect labrum.

DEBRIDEMENT, REPAIR, RECONSTRUCTION: IT PROBABLY MATTERS

Although there are those who can tolerate an imperfect labrum, there are clearly those who cannot. Aside from the clinical data that show fairly convincingly the superiority of labral restoration to debridement, there are in vivo studies that offer some rationale as why this may be.

The Labrum is a Pain Generator

Haversath and colleagues[18] reported that there is pain-associated free nerve expression within the labrum, predominately at its base with the highest concentration anterosuperiorly.

The Labrum is a Fibrocartilaginous Structure

Seldes and colleagues[19] described the histology of the labrum as a cartilaginous structure similar to a meniscus. The knee literature shows good results with repair of certain types of acute meniscal tears,[20] but notably bad results with repair of complex, degenerative meniscal tears.[21,22] Although not completely analogous structures, it would be difficult to imagine that a complex degenerative tear of a fibrocartilaginous structure in the hip would heal at a markedly higher rate by placing sutures around it. Furthermore, Haemer and colleagues[23] demonstrated that degeneration and tearing of the labrum leads to increased permeability resulting in loss of fluid support and increased consolidation rate of the articular cartilage in a finite element model.

Biomechanical Function Can Be Restored Through Repair or Reconstruction

Biomechanical studies have pointed to at least partial restoration of time zero hip biomechanics after a repair or reconstruction of a compromised labrum. In a cadaveric model, Nepple and colleagues[24] found labral reconstruction and repair significantly improved stability to distractive forces compared with labral resection, as well as improving intra-articular fluid pressurization compared with labral tear and partial resection conditions. Interestingly, they also found that labral reconstruction outperformed labral repair in improving fluid pressurization and maintaining it over time.[3] Similarly, Lee and colleagues[25] found that while segmental anterosuperior labral resection resulted in significantly decreased contact areas and increased contact pressures, these areas and pressures were partially restored by labral reconstruction.

AUTHOR'S TREATMENT ALGORITHM FOR LABRAL MANAGEMENT

Based on the previously described evidence and the author's personal experience, this is the treatment algorithm I currently use (**Fig. 1**, **Table 2**). Surgeons should select the appropriate treatment for any individual patient based on their own experience with the procedure and what they feel will offer the patient the best chance at a good outcome.

- *Labral debridement*
  - Peripheral tear of the without instability at its base
    - Labrum must be of functional size after debridement
  - Labrum is damaged beyond repair and a reconstruction is not possible.

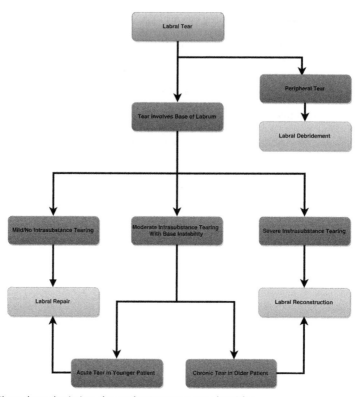

Fig. 1. Flow chart depicting the author's treatment algorithm.

- ○ Favored when the pathology and pain generation do not appear to be of labral origin
- Labral repair
  - ○ The labral base is unstable or detached
  - ○ Intrasubstance tearing is mild or moderate
- Labral reconstruction
  - ○ Segmental labral defect
  - ○ Severe intrasubstance damage (**Fig. 2**)

Table 2 Surgical considerations for labral treatment	Restores Anatomic Function	Removes Pain-Generating Tissue	Technical Complexity	Long-Term Follow-up Studies Exist
Labral debridement	Low[a]	High	Low	Medium
Labral repair	High	Low[c]	High	Medium
Labral reconstruction	High[b]	Very High	Very High	Low

[a] If insufficient labral tissue remains after debridement.
[b] If appropriately tensioned circumferential seal is restored.
[c] If sufficient intact labral tissue remains, this can be repaired following debridement of damaged pain-generating tissue.

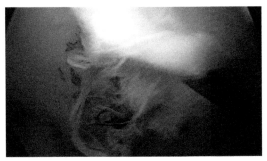

Fig. 2. Labrum with severe intrasubstance damage in a 24-year-old male hockey player with severe CAM type FAI.

- ○ Diminutive labral remnant after debridement
  - ■ Insufficient labral tissue is considered to be less than 2 to 3 mm because it lacks the surface area to heal and repair may not create a sufficient fluid seal[26]
- ○ Favored in revision of failed labral repair

Controversial Indications for Labral Reconstruction

Revision hip arthroscopy
In a patient who has undergone a previous hip arthroscopy either with a labral debridement or repair, it is often the case in which the labral tissue is compromised. Similarly, it is at times unclear at the time of arthroscopy what the cause or causes of the failure of the previous procedure are. As the labrum itself can be a pain generator, resection and reconstruction can be a useful tool to remove damaged pain-generating tissue and replace it with aneural tissue of better quality and better mechanical properties. Additionally, resection of the labrum provides unlimited access to the rim of the acetabulum to correct any bony or chondral irregularity that may be present but "hidden" beneath the labrum.

Labral tears with moderate intrasubstance damage
In patients with moderate intrasubstance damage and instability at the base of the labrum, there are several factors that can be considered in the decision of whether to repair or reconstruct the labrum:

a. Younger patients are more likely to heal a repair than older patients. I favor reconstruction in older patients.
b. More acute tears are more likely to heal than chronic tears. I favor repair in more acute settings.
c. Severe CAM-type FAI if corrected will likely provide a favorable environment for labral healing. I favor repair in these settings.
d. Intrasubstance synovitic changes or fatty changes (as often seen with paralabral cysts on MRI) likely indicate a more advanced degree and chronicity of tissue compromise. I favor reconstruction in these settings.

Coxa Profunda Pincer Deformities
Coxa profunda deformities often are accompanied by (or caused by) ossification of the labrum (particularly posteriorly). In these cases, to adequately correct the deformity, a labral resection must be performed. I will then perform a labral reconstruction. In cases in which the labrum has not ossified but there is a deformity that requires a labral

takedown and a substantial osteoplasty of the acetabular rim, the labral tissue will often not fit appropriately onto the recessed acetabular rim or will be damaged in the process of removing it. Additionally, in these cases, access to the rim is markedly easier and more thorough if the labrum is entirely resected.

SURGICAL TECHNIQUES
Labral Debridement and Repair

Step by step description of procedure

After the patient is positioned, prepped, and draped as described elsewhere, the following steps are undertaken:

- Traction is applied.
- The distracted hip is visualized fluoroscopically; approximately 10 mm of joint space is typically adequate.
- A spinal needle is used to set the anterolateral portal. This is typically placed approximately 1 cm anterior and superior to the tip of the greater trochanter, but should be adjusted so as to have a useful portal that does not penetrate the labrum or scuff the femoral head. This is visualized fluoroscopically to ensure optimal position.
- A Seldinger technique is used to create an anterolateral portal using a nitinol wire passed through the spinal needle that is then removed. An arthroscopic cannula is then placed over this guidewire.
- The camera is inserted into the joint. *At this point, no arthroscopic fluid is used as there is no outflow portal.*
- A spinal needle is then used to localize the mid anterior portal, which is placed at approximately the midpoint, in the medial-lateral plane between the tip of the greater trochanter and the antero-superior iliac spine and approximately 7 cm distal to the anterolateral portal. *The placement of this portal is variable and dependent on anatomy. Fluoroscopy is of limited utility. In general, if you are having trouble, consider that this portal is placed much more in-line with your antero-lateral portal than you might think. There are commercially available devices to help with placement of this portal, but these are of questionable value. Practice and familiarity with the procedure are your best tools.*
- Typically the next step is to perform a capsulotomy connecting the anterolateral and midanterior portals. This is done with a banana knife or beaver blade. *This step is occasionally unnecessary in patients in whom peripheral compartment work is not indicated and/or patients in whom instability is an issue. When performing the capsulotomy, be sure to leave a sufficient capsule on the acetabular side so that it may be repaired at the end of the procedure.*
- At this point, the entire central compartment is visible and should be inspected and the labrum should be probed to assess for tears and instability.
- If a labral tear is encountered, it should then be assessed for extent and whether it is amenable to repair. Tears with instability at the base should be repaired. Peripheral fraying of the labrum should be debrided. *In patients with complex degenerative tears with significant intrasubstance tearing and synovitis, consideration should be given to resection and reconstruction (see previously).*

Labral debridement

- If labral debridement is indicated, this is performed with an arthroscopic shaver, an electrocautery, and/or an arthroscopic biter.
- The base of the labrum should be left intact if possible.

Labral repair
- If a labral repair is performed, the next step is to identify the acetabular rim to which the labrum is usually still at least partially attached.
- The bone of the acetabulum is exposed with a shaver and/or an electrocautery device with careful attention paid to labral preservation.
- If there is significant damage at the chondro-labral junction, or a significant acetabuloplasty is to be performed based on preoperative imaging demonstrating significant pincer-type FAI, then burring of the acetabular rim is undertaken to effect an appropriate pincer correction or to eliminate the area of damage at the chondro-labral junction. *DO NOT OVER-RESECT THE ACETABULAR RIM, AS THIS WILL DESTABILIZE THE HIP.*
- Burring is then undertaken to correct the bony aspect of the pathology.
- Damaged labrum and damaged and/or redundant articular cartilage is then resected with an arthroscopic biter, shaver, and/or electrocautery device.
- If there is no detachment or significant damage on the articular side of the chondro-labral junction and there is no need for a significant acetabuloplasty, the chondro-labral junction may be preserved. In this case, burring is performed only to the extent necessary to get to a surface of bleeding bone for labral repair/refixation.
- Place anchors into the acetabular rim.
  - This can be done through either of the existing portals, or through a distal anterolateral (DALA) portal localized with a spinal needle and placed approximately 5 to 8 cm distal to the anterolateral portal.
  - It is often easier to place all of the anchors at one time and then proceed to the repair, as the acetabulum is most exposed at this time.
  - The drill guide should be positioned as close as possible to the acetabular rim to effect anatomic repair.
  - The surgeon should consider drilling these holes himself for the purposes of tactile feedback while the assistant holds the camera focused on the acetabular articular surface to ensure that there is no violation of same.
  - Similarly, the holes for anchor placement should not violate the extra-articular portion of the bone either, particularly anteriorly as the bone is thin in this area and a protruding anchor can be an irritant to the psoas tendon.
    - Perforation through the extra-articular side of the acetabulum can be checked by palpation with a nitinol wire
- Place a clear cannula for suture management into the midanterior portal.
- Retrieve the post suture limb from the anterior-most suture anchor.
- Pass the other suture limb from the most anterior anchor through the chondro-labral junction.
- Grasp this suture limb and retrieve it through the cannula. It is at this point when the surgeon must decide whether to use a simple loop suture or a vertical mattress (also known as a "base-refixation suture")[26] (see **Fig. 2**).
  - Although I prefer the vertical mattress configuration in most settings, I feel that the anatomy of the patient's labrum ought to dictate the suture configuration.
    - For more cylindrical and smaller labra, a simple loop suture is preferable.
    - For more hypertrophic and/or meniscoid labra, a vertical mattress is preferable to restore the original anatomic configuration (**Figs. 3** and **4**).
    - Sutures are then tied using standard arthroscopic knot tying technique. In large etched tears, it can be beneficial to use an arthroscopic grasper placed through the distal accessory portal to hold appropriate tension on the labrum during suture fixation.

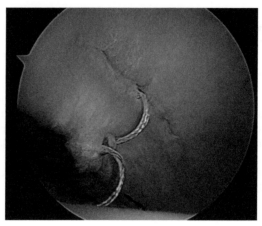

Fig. 3. Suture retrieval through the labrum for a vertical mattress stitch configuration.

- *Alternatively, the sutures for labral repair can be placed first and then passed through knotless anchors that are then placed into the acetabular rim.*

LABRAL RECONSTRUCTION PREFERRED TECHNIQUE AND RATIONALE

Although labral reconstruction likely offers a superior solution for certain difficult labral problems, the difference in some patients between a repair/debridement and a reconstruction may be marginal. It is imperative that the surgeon undertake this procedure with careful consideration of the significant technical difficulty and narrow margin for error in patients who are otherwise young and healthy. Likewise, it is incumbent on each individual surgeon to decide whether, in their hands, the increased risk and length of the procedure is likely to be of meaningful benefit to the patient.

There are a wide variety of techniques and graft choices used in the literature on labral reconstruction. There is no high-level evidence to distinguish between these

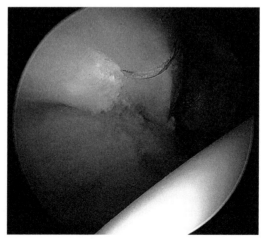

Fig. 4. Labral fixation showing a looped suture at a more circumferential portion of the labrum and a vertical mattress suture configuration at a more meniscoid portion of the labrum father anteriorly.

techniques and graft choices. Thus, surgeons are left to decide what they are most comfortable with based on their experience, the goals they are trying to accomplish, and their comfort level with accessing the far-reaches of the acetabulum. The 2 main choices in labral reconstruction are length of reconstruction and graft choice.

Length of Reconstruction: Longer is Better

Much of the labral reconstruction literature, both biomechanical and clinical, reflects use of relatively short grafts of 3 to 4 cm that reconstruct typically the anterosuperior portion of the labrum. Although these results are encouraging, it has been my personal experience[16] as well as that reported by White and colleagues[13] that longer grafts fare better. The likely reasons for this are twofold:

1. Segmental grafts have 2 junction points with the native labrum in high-stress areas. Restoring the hoop stress stability of the labral seal at 2 high-stress points with side-to-side fixation is a technical challenge to reproducibly achieve. A circumferential labral graft (as described later in this article) has either no junction points or one far posteroinferiorly at an area of low stress.
2. The labrum is a known pain generator. Resecting more labral tissue results in greater pain relief, as long as stability is also restored.

Graft Choice

The choice of graft is probably less important than the length and technique of the reconstruction. The demands on a labral graft or native labrum are that it must act as a collagen scaffold for integration onto the acetabular rim and that it must be strong enough to withstand the forces across it. The forces to which a labrum is subjected are far exceeded by those of other structures that are routinely reconstructed with grafts around the body. Thus, although the literature on graft choice in anterior cruciate ligament (ACL) reconstruction shows a trend toward higher failure rates in allografts than in autografts, with its high torsional and tensile demands, the ACL is hardly an analogous structure to the acetabular labrum, thus this failure rate is likely not applicable.

The autograft choices that have been described are ligamentum teres in an open approach[10] (not a feasible arthroscopic choice), iliotibial band,[11] and hamstring.[12,13] Although not disqualifying, each of these grafts carries increased surgical site morbidity, a cosmetic cost and an increase in operative time relative to an allograft.

Whether the graft is an autograft or allograft, the tissue choices are similar. I have used anterior tibialis, posterior tibialis, semitendinosus and fascia lata allografts, and iliotibial band autografts. In my experience, the most consistent grafts can be made from fascia lata allografts. Using my preferred technique, the graft is tubularized using absorbable sutures to a size of 6 mm × 90 to 100 mm (**Fig. 5**).

Technique

- The native labrum is resected from the transverse acetabular ligament anteroinferiorly to the 8 o'clock position posteroinferiorly.
  - To access the anteroinferior acetabular rim, it is preferable to incise a small portion of the iliofemoral ligament adjacent to the psoas fossa instead of

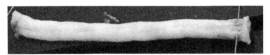

Fig. 5. 90 × 6 mm graft for labral reconstruction from fascia lata allograft following tubularization using multiple absorbable braided sutures.

extending the capsulotomy through this important stabilizing portion of ligament.
- ○ Alternatively, the anteroinferior labrum and rim can be easily accessed with the hip out of traction and in approximately 40° of flexion.
- The rim of the acetabulum is burred throughout the length of the proposed reconstruction. Acetabular osteoplasty is performed if necessary.
  - ○ Posteroinferiorly, the rim is burred behind the labrum to approximately the 7:30 position while the labral remnant is left intact in this area. This allows fixation of the graft to the labrum in an area of low stress and obviates the need for cutting excess graft, as any excess is minimal and is fixated outside of the native labrum.
  - ○ The posteroinferior labrum is usually undamaged. If this is not the case, the labrum should be resected to the transverse acetabular ligament posteroinferiorly. In this situation, excess graft may need to be excised.
- Through the DALA portal, anchors are placed around the rim with the exception of the posteroinferior anchor (**Fig. 6**).
  - ○ All anchors should be positioned as close to the articular surface as possible without violation of same so as to achieve restoration of suction seal by the labral graft.
  - ○ The anteroinferior anchor(s) are sometimes more easily placed through the midanterior portal. If this is the case, it is more efficient to place these through the cannula just before passage of the graft.
- The posteroinferior anchor is placed at approximately the 7:30 position behind the labral remnant.
- The lead suture from the posteroinferior anchor is passed in a vertical mattress fashion through the native labral remnant and tagged for future passage through the posterior portion of the graft.
- Sutures from all anchors are retrieved through the anterolateral portal to keep them out of the way.
- A clear cannula is placed through the mid anterior portal and the sutures from the anteroinferior anchor are retrieved through this portal.

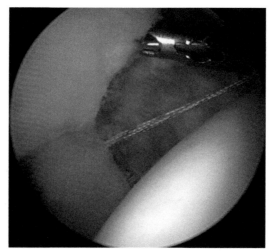

Fig. 6. Placement of third anchor through DALA portal. Camera is in anterolateral portal. Sutures from first anchor are visible anteroinferiorly and from second in the iliopsoas fossa.

- The lead suture limb is weaved through the end of the graft.
- The post suture limb is pulled to draw the graft into the cannula while the graft is gently pushed down the cannula by a blunt device until the graft is fully in the joint.
  - Tension should be kept on the sutures from the other anchors during graft passage to avoid tangles.
- Once the graft is positioned on the rim of the acetabulum anteroinferiorly, the suture that the graft has been passed down is tied and then cut.
- The sutures from the second suture anchor are then retrieved through the cannula, and passed around and/or through the graft.
- Through the DALA portal, a blunt grasper is used to manipulate and tension the graft on the acetabular rim. It is held in the desired position with the desired tension by an assistant while the suture is tied.
- This process is repeated sequentially across the rim of the acetabulum, proceeding anteriorly to posteriorly.
  - Typically at approximately the 12 o'clock position, the clear cannula needs to be moved to the DALA portal and the camera to the mid anterior portal with graft manipulation taking place through the anterolateral portal
- For the posteroinferior suture, the limb that was previously passed through the native labrum now should be passed through the graft. This should be done in an area of the graft that will appropriately tension the graft so that it lies circumferentially on the rim and is not overtensioned or undertensioned.
  - Once this suture is passed at the optimal spot on the graft, the sutures are retrieved and tied through the cannula. The post suture should be free and the lead suture should be in a vertical mattress through the labrum and the graft so that when this suture is tied, appropriate tension is achieved, the graft and the labrum are lying opposed with the graft and any remaining length situated extra-articularly (**Fig. 7**).
- At this point, the labral graft is probed throughout. It is not uncommon to find spots that need extra fixation. Additional anchors should be placed in these spots and sutures passed and tied as in a labral repair.

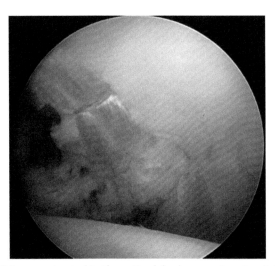

Fig. 7. Labral graft is approximated to the native labral remnant posteroinferiorly. There is a contiguous seal established with excess graft remaining extra-articularly.

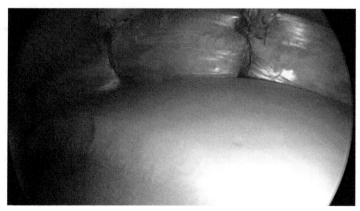

Fig. 8. Dynamic examination following labral reconstruction with reestablishment of seal on femoral head.

- The hip is then taken out of traction and a dynamic examination is performed to ensure restoration of suction seal and lack of impingement (**Fig. 8**).

POSTOPERATIVE CARE

For labral debridement, labral repair, and labral reconstruction, patients have protected weight-bearing with crutches for typically 2 to 4 weeks until their gait has normalized. I do not restrict patients differentially based on how the labral treatment performed. It is not unusual for patients undergoing a circumferential reconstruction to feel very little pain very quickly. It is imperative that these patients are instructed to take it slowly regardless of how they feel.

Weight-bearing will be more restricted for greater duration of time based on concomitant procedures (eg, chondral restorative procedure, capsular plication, gluteal tendon repair). Passive motion is begun immediately either with a continuous passive motion machine or with a stationary bike without resistance.

Time to initiation of physical therapy is variable, but is usually within 3 to 4 days. Gentle range of motion and isometric exercises are begun in the early phases with progression to more active strengthening focused on the core and gluteal musculature, and establishing a normal gait pattern as weeks progress. Manual therapy can be a valuable adjunct during the recovery phase.

Depending on the goals and rate of progress of the patient, a gradual return to running can begin at 10 to 12 weeks. Although some investigators have reported successful return to competitive athletics as early as 3 months, most advocate a minimum of 4 to 6 months, particularly for high hip-demand sports, such as football, lacrosse, soccer, ballet, or wrestling. For more information, see Malloy P, Gray K, Wolff AB: Rehabilitation After Hip Arthroscopy: A Movement Control-Based Perspective, in this issue. Videos and full protocols also are available at www.andrewwolffmd.com.

SUMMARY

Indications for treatment of hip labral pathology are in evolution. On the one hand, there are individuals who can tolerate a severely damaged or missing labrum, while on the other there are those whose hip function is severely compromised due to labral imperfection. Given the difficulty distinguishing between these patients, the goal with arthroscopic hip surgery should be to restore the labral anatomy to approximate that of a normal hip and to remove pain-generating irreparable labral tissue. With those goals in mind, debridement, repair, and reconstruction all can be of utility in the treatment of hip labral pathology.

REFERENCES

1. Ferguson SJ, Bryant JT, Ganz R, et al. An in vitro investigation of the acetabular labral seal in hip joint mechanics. J Biomech 2003;36(2):171–8.
2. Ferguson SJ, Bryant JT, Ganz R, et al. The influence of the acetabular labrum on hip joint cartilage consolidation: a poroelastic finite element model. J Biomech 2000;33(8):953–60.
3. Philippon MJ, Nepple JJ, Campbell KJ, et al. The hip fluid seal–part I: the effect of an acetabular labral tear, repair, resection, and reconstruction on hip stability to distraction. Knee Surg Sports Traumatol Arthrosc 2014;22:722–9.
4. Soltz MA, Ateshian GA. Experimental verification and theoretical prediction of cartilage interstitial fluid pressurization at an impermeable contact interface in confined compression. J Biomech 1998;31(10):927–34.
5. Song Y, Ito H, Kourtis L, et al. Articular cartilage friction increases in hip joints after the removal of acetabular labrum. J Biomech 2012;45(3):524–30.
6. Espinosa N, Rothenfluh DA, Beck M, et al. Treatment of femoro-acetabular impingement: preliminary results of labral re-fixation. J Bone Joint Surg Am 2006;88:925–35.
7. Larson CM, Giveans MR. Arthroscopic debridement versus refixation of the acetabular labrum associated with femoroacetabular impingement. Arthroscopy 2009;25(4):369–76.
8. Larson CM, Giveans MR, Stone RM. Arthroscopic debridement versus refixation of the acetabular labrum associated with femoroacetabular impingement: mean 3.5 year follow-up. Am J Sports Med 2012;40(5):1015–21.
9. Philippon MJ, Briggs KK, Yen YM, et al. Outcomes following hip arthroscopy for femoroacetabular impingement with associated chondrolabral dysfunction: minimum two-year follow-up. J Bone Joint Surg Br 2009;91(1):16–23.
10. Sierra RJ, Trousdale RT. Labral reconstruction using the ligamentum teres capitis: report of a new technique. Clin Orthop Relat Res 2009;467(3):753–9.
11. Philippon MJ, Briggs KK, Hay CJ, et al. Arthroscopic labral reconstruction in the hip using iliotibial band autograft: technique and early outcomes. Arthroscopy 2010;26(6):750–6.
12. Geyer MF, Philippon MJ, Fagrelius TS, et al. Acetabular labral reconstruction with an iliotibial band autograft: outcome and survivorship analysis at minimum 3-year follow-up. Am J Sports Med 2013;41:1750–6.
13. White BJ, Stapleford AB, Hawkes TK, et al. Allograft use in arthroscopic labral reconstruction of the hip with front-to-back fixation technique: minimum 2-year follow-up. Arthroscopy 2015;32(1):26–32.
14. Domb BG, El Bita YF, Stake CE, et al. Arthroscopic labral reconstruction is superior to segmental resection for irreparable labral tears in the hip: a matched-pair controlled study with minimum 2-year follow-up. Am J Sports Med 2014;42(1):122–30.
15. Matsuda DK, Burchette RJ. Arthroscopic hip labral reconstruction with a gracilis autograft versus labral refixation: 2-year minimum outcomes. Am J Sports Med 2013;41(5):980–7.

16. Wolff A, Hogan G, Napoli A. Arthroscopic circumferential acetabular labral reconstruction using fascia lata allograft: one-year patient reported outcomes. ISHA Annual Scientific Meeting Podium Presentation. Cambridge University, Cambridge, September 25, 2015.

17. Register B, Pennock AT, Ho CP, et al. Prevalence of abnormal hip findings in asymptomatic participants: a prospective, blinded study. Am J Sports Med 2012;40(12):2720–4.

18. Haversath M, Hanke J, Landgraeber S, et al. The distribution of nociceptive innervation in the painful hip: a histological investigation. Bone Joint J 2013;95B(6): 770–6.

19. Seldes RM, Tan V, Hunt J, et al. Anatomy, histologic features, and vascularity of the adult acetabular labrum. Clin Orthop Relat Res 2001;382:232–40.

20. Henning CE. Current status of meniscus salvage. Clin Sports Med 1990;9(3): 567–76.

21. Herrlin S, Hållander M, Wange P, et al. Arthroscopic or conservative treatment of degenerative medial meniscal tears: a prospective randomised trial. Knee Surg Sports Traumatol Arthrosc 2007;15(4):393–401.

22. Katz JN, Brophy RH, Chaisson CE, et al. Surgery versus physical therapy for a meniscal tear and osteoarthritis. N Engl J Med 2013;368(18):1675–84.

23. Haemer JM, Carter DR, Giori NJ. The low permeability of healthy meniscus and labrum limit articular cartilage consolidation and maintain fluid load support in the knee and hip. J Biomech 2012;45(8):1450–6.

24. Nepple JJ, Philippon MJ, Campbell KJ, et al. The hip fluid seal–part II: the effect of an acetabular labral tear, repair, resection, and reconstruction on hip stability to distraction. Knee Surg Sports Traumatol Arthrosc 2014;22:730–6.

25. Lee S, Wuerz TH, Shewman E, et al. Labral reconstruction with iliotibial band autografts and semitendinosus allografts improves hip joint contact area and contact pressure: an in vitro analysis. Am J Sports Med 2015;43:98–104.

26. Fry R, Domb B. Labral base refixation in the hip: rationale and technique for an anatomic approach to labral repair. Arthroscopy 2010;26(9):10.

Chondral Lesions of the Hip

Zachariah S. Logan, MD[a], John M. Redmond, MD[a,b], Sarah C. Spelsberg, PA-C[a],
Timothy J. Jackson, MD[b,c], Benjamin G. Domb, MD[b,d],*

KEYWORDS

- Chondral injuries • Treatment options • Labral damage • Cartilage injuries

KEY POINTS

- The treatment of chondral injuries in the hip is challenging and frequently accompanies labral damage.
- Chondroplasty, microfracture, osteochondral graft transfers, and autologous chondrocyte implantation are available treatment options.
- Chondroplasty and microfracture procedures can be performed arthroscopically, whereas osteochondral graft transfers and autologous chondrocyte implantation require an open surgical hip dislocation for exposure.

The treatment of chondral injuries in the hip is challenging. As the understanding of the hip joint continues to evolve, effective treatment strategies are emerging. Conditions such as femoroacetabular impingement (FAI), acetabular dysplasia, trauma, and avascular necrosis (AVN) frequently involve damage to the chondral surface and subsequent clinical symptoms in young adults. Several studies have documented a high prevalence of chondral injuries encountered when performing hip arthroscopy for FAI and dysplasia.[1,2] A thorough understanding of chondral injuries encountered during hip preservation is helpful for preoperative planning and intraoperative treatment.

Several chondral damage classification systems have been proposed[3–5] (**Table 1**). These classification systems, along with the size of the defect, can be used to guide treatment decisions. McCarthy and Lee[1] reported on 457 arthroscopic examinations of the hip and found that 59% of their patients had damage in the anterior quadrant

Disclosures: Dr B.G. Domb is a board member at the American Hip Institute and The AANA Learning Center Committee; is a paid consultant for Amplitude, Arthrex, Pacira, and Stryker; and receives royalties from Arthrex, Djo Global, and Orthomerica. The American Hip Institute receives research support from Arthrex, ATI, Breg, Pacira, and Stryker. No other authors have anything to disclose.
[a] Department of Orthopaedics, Mayo Clinic Florida, 4500 San Pablo Road South, Jacksonville, FL 32224, USA; [b] American Hip Institute, Westmont, IL, USA; [c] Orthopedic Medical Associates, Pasadena, CA, USA; [d] Hinsdale Orthopaedics, Hinsdale, IL, USA
* Corresponding author. American Hip Institute, Westmont, IL.
E-mail address: DrDomb@americanhipinstitute.org

Table 1
Articular injury classifications

Classification	Grade	Features
Outerbridge[4]	0	Normal-appearing cartilage
	1	Soft, swollen cartilage
	2	Partial-thickness defect, or with diameter <1.5 cm
	3	Fissures that extend to the subchondral surface with diameter >1.5 cm
	4	Exposed subchondral bone
Beck et al[3]	0	Normal; macroscopically sound cartilage
	1	Malacia; roughening of surface, fibrillations
	2	Pitting malacia; rough, thin with deep fissuring to the bone
	3	Debonding; normal-appearing cartilage that has lost subchondral fixation
	4	Cleavage; thin, frayed cartilage that has lost subchondral fixation
	5	Defect; full-thickness defect
ALAD[5]	1	Softening of the adjacent cartilage
	2	Early peel-back of the cartilage
	3	Large flap of cartilage
	4	Cartilage loss

Abbreviation: ALAD, acetabular labrum articular disruption.

of the acetabulum and were associated with labral disorder. This finding is expected given that the proposed mechanisms of FAI and dysplasia predominantly cause stress on the anterosuperior acetabulum.

Understanding of hip joint biomechanics continues to grow. Investigators have proposed several important functions of the acetabular labral tissue, and have described its role in the development of acetabular chondral disorders. An intact labrum is required to prevent extravasation of the water content of acetabular cartilage. The labrum maintains the intra-articular fluid hydrostatic pressure, allowing the femoral head to, in effect, float on the surface of the cartilage. Loss of the labral seal integrity allows extravasation of the joint fluid, thereby increasing the stresses of the resultant cartilage contact.

Another mechanism by which the labrum may decrease the compression of the cartilage layers and help prevent their injury is because of its microanatomy. The labrum is largely made of dense fibrocartilage and collagen types I and III. This labrum acts as a stopper valve for the interstitial fluid content of the proteoglycan-rich acetabular cartilage, with which the labrum is anatomically continuous, and prevents the consolidation of the articular cartilage layers. Disruption of the labrum may lead to chondral injury.

The evidence to support treatment of chondral injuries in the hip lags behind the understanding of the knee.[6] However, with techniques such as open surgical hip dislocation and hip arthroscopy the same techniques used in the knee may be applied to the hip. This article describes the clinical presentation of chondral injuries and the modalities available to treat them.

CLINICAL PRESENTATION

The clinical presentations of hip disorders that lead to chondral damage are variable. Femoroacetabular impingement, dysplasia, acetabular osteochondritis dissecans lesions, or femoral AVN can all result in hip pain significant enough to seek orthopedic consultation.[7–10] A thorough history and physical examination is necessary, coupled with appropriate imaging techniques, to elucidate the problem and guide treatment. Although this seems intuitive, patients with FAI see an average of 4.2 providers and wait 3 years for a diagnosis. Thirteen percent have undergone surgery that did not address the underlying hip disorder.[7] It is important to recognize that chondral damage may be an effect, not a cause.[10]

Impingement

Femoroacetabular impingement presents most often with a complaint of dull achy groin pain on the affected side. It is typically caused by cam (femoral) or pincer (acetabular) deformities, either alone or in combination.[7,8] Patients often show the C sign (placing the hand cupped in a C shape around the proximal femur) indicating pain deep in the hip.[9] They may complain of increased pain after sitting for long periods. On physical examination, the anterior impingement sign is positive (the hip and knee are flexed to 90°; the thigh is adducted and internally rotated). Hip flexion and internal rotation can be limited or decreased.[8] Correct imaging is necessary to differentiate between cam and pincer causes.[7-10] The biomechanics and subsequent disorders of cam and pincer hip morphologies vary greatly. Cam impingement typically causes damage to the anterosuperior acetabulum, whereas a pincer lesion causes more circumferential damage in a narrow ring of acetabular cartilage.[10] Patients with cam deformity of the hip frequently have delamination of the anterosuperior chondral surface of the acetabulum. These lesions can be extensive at a young age and are challenging to treat.

Hip Dysplasia

Hip dysplasia often first presents with pain and/or a limp in an adolescent or young adult. Patients are frequently female and show excessive hip motion. Note that the physical findings and presentation evolve during development. The dysplastic hip joint morphology results in abnormal loading of the acetabular rim, which leads to chondrolabral disorder. The extent of osteochondral damage is contingent on the deformity, loading pattern, and patient activity.[11]

Avascular Necrosis

AVN of the femoral head can vary in presentation secondary to the location of the lesion. The cause varies and includes Perthes, alcohol abuse, smoking, and steroid use as risk factors.[12-14] It is initially painless and as the disease progresses patients begin to have pain. It is most commonly groin pain; however, patients may also complain of pain in the buttock, knee, or greater trochanter. Pain is made worse with weight bearing and better with rest. Patients have progressively limited range of motion. On physical examination, patients have pain with internal rotation and straight leg raise against resistance, and the log roll test (passive internal and external rotation of the leg in extension) is painful if the condition includes capsular synovitis. Passive abduction is often limited. Early disease typically only involves the femur and attempts at chondral preservation are feasible.

TREATMENT
Chondroplasty

Chondroplasty is a frequently performed technique for partial-thickness chondral injuries at the time of hip arthroscopy. It is performed in conjunction with acetabular labral treatment, and as such there are no published series of isolated acetabular chondroplasties in the literature. However, during arthroscopic evaluation and treatment of the hip, the chondral surface frequently has areas that are treated with chondroplasty to avoid unstable chondral flaps. No special equipment is needed. Previous investigators have shown this to be a satisfactory treatment strategy for low-grade/partial-thickness chondral injures.[15]

Microfracture

Microfracture is a commonly used technique for the treatment of small chondral defects in the knee. Used for the appropriate indication (ie, unipolar defects smaller than 4 cm^2), results are favorable.[15,16] There is currently less evidence regarding its use in the hip,[2,17–19] and this is even more apparent for femoral lesions than for acetabular lesions. The performance of the microfracture proceeds in a similar fashion as it would in the knee, as shown in **Fig. 1**. The loose portions of the chondral flap are debrided sharply back to stable cartilage with perpendicular walls. The base of the defect is roughened. Either chondral picks or specialty drills[20] can then be used to perpendicularly perforate the central bed with 3-mm holes spaced about 3 mm apart. These holes should be deep enough to puncture the subchondral bone and release marrow contents, which can then creep out into the defect, filling it with the growth factors needed for the resultant fibrocartilage formation.[21] Several investigators have examined both the structural and functional results of microfracture.[15,19,22] Philippon and colleagues[22] examined whether acetabular defects responded to microfracture by producing reparative fibrocartilage on second-look arthroscopies in a group of 9 patients. The average fill of the defects was 91%. The function of this repair was not evaluated with outcome measurements.[22] Byrd and Jones[23] reported on 9 patients who had grade 4 chondral lesions, presumably from an inverted acetabular labrum. Three of these patients had small, well-circumscribed lesions that were treated with microfracture; these were the only patients who returned to sports activities at 2 years.[23] In a subset of their 207 patients who underwent arthroscopic management of FAI, Byrd and Jones[24] later reported an improvement in the Modified Harris Hip Score in 58 patients who received microfracture for their grade 4 lesions. At 2-year follow-up, scores had improved from 65 to 85.[24] As might be predicted, the likelihood of success of microfracture declines with increasing arthritis.[25,26]

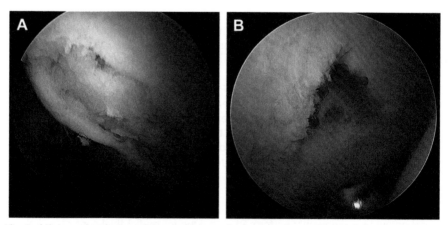

Fig. 1. (*A*) A grade 4 lesion of the cartilage surface of the femoral head, following debridement of any unstable cartilage. This defect is now contained, with a rim of healthy, stable cartilage, ready for subchondral perforation with a microfracture technique. (*B*) A similar lesion, following performance of microfracture, with visual seepage of the marrow contents that will ultimately lead to fibrocartilage formation.

Microfracture is not a technically demanding procedure to perform. It is also low cost, as there is little additional instrumentation required. Although there have been limitations with the studies evaluating the effectiveness of microfracture for hip lesions, including small sample sizes and a lack of appropriate control groups, the short-term results have been favorable in patients who do not have advanced arthritis. Longer-term studies are needed to better define the role of microfracture in treating hip cartilage lesions.

Osteochondral Allograft Transplantation

In larger osteochondral defects of the hip, osteochondral allograft transplant (OATS) has had good clinical results. Indications are borrowed from the knee literature. Patients with signs of osteoarthritis (OA) are not good candidates, nor are those that are older than 50 years. It can be used in those instances in which defects penetrate the subchondral layers, or have an area larger than 2.5 to 3 cm^2.[27,28] From a technical standpoint, these lesions can be challenging to treat with other methods. For instance, finding enough expendable healthy cartilage to fill these voids as well as the time required to drill a grid and shape an array of plugs precludes the use of mosaicplasty. Lesions of this size outstrip the ability of the fibrocartilage resulting from microfracture to provide an acceptable clinical result. Rather than using the numerous recipient holes of mosaicplasty, OATS is performed by consolidating the total area into 1 plug, harvested from a cadaveric allograft, which is then inset in a similar fashion with an attempt to maintain articular surface geometry. The sequence of OATS is shown in **Fig. 2**. Its use in the hip was first described by Meyers[29] in the mid-1980s. There were 25 patients in whom the technique was performed, 20 of whom had postcollapse AVN and 1 who sustained a femoral head fracture-dislocation. In those patients who had steroid-induced osteonecrosis, the failure rate was 50%. In those patients who did not, the failure rate was 20%. Krych and colleagues[27] used OATS in 2 patients

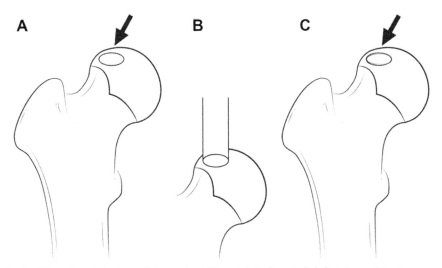

Fig. 2. Osteochondral allograft transplantation. (*A*) A chondral defect (*arrow*) is shown on the femoral head. (*B*) The osteochondral allograft is harvested from a donor femoral head using a harvesting cylinder. (*C*) The defect (*arrow*) is filled with the harvested osteochondral allograft.

to manage acetabular-sided defects. An acetabular allograft was used. One patient had a periacetabular cyst and the other fibrous dysplasia, treated with curettage and cementing. At 2 years, the first patient had a Modified Harris Hip Score (MHHS) improvement from 75 to 97, and the second patient from 79 to 100, at 3 years.

OATS has its flaws. There is a risk of transmission of disease. Cadaveric allograft relies on donors and is occasionally scarce, and the steps of graft harvest, processing, and storage can be complex.[27]

Autologous Chondrocyte Implantation/Matrix-assisted Autologous Chondrocyte Implantation

Autologous chondrocyte implantation (ACI) is performed in a 2-stage fashion. Healthy chondrocytes are harvested from a remote joint and cultivated ex vivo. Once these have increased in number sufficient to fill the defect, they are then injected underneath a patch graft sewn to the surrounding cartilage, which can be a synthetic material or a periosteal autograft. In the hip, this can be a particularly challenging procedure and requires surgical dislocation for complete access to perform the implantation. Inherent in this is the risk of AVN. Ganz and colleagues[30] described a technique to limit the occurrence of AVN following surgical hip dislocation. There were no patients in a cohort of 213 who subsequently developed AVN. Matrix-assisted ACI (MACI) can be done without the need for a graft. MACI relies on a biodegradable substrate on which the chondrocytes are implanted. This implantation can be completed without the need for an open dislocation.[31] Reports on its use are favorable. Akimau and colleagues[32] used ACI in a case of late femoral head AVN that developed after fracture-dislocation and initial treatment with open reduction with internal fixation 21 months earlier. A collagen patch was used to cover the femoral head after bone grafting the subchondral defects. Chondrocytes were injected underneath the patch. A biopsy was later done that showed a 2-mm cap of predominantly fibrocartilage, although there were some small areas of hyaline-appearing tissue.[32] At final follow-up of 12 months, his Harris Hip Score (HHS) had improved to 76 from 52. Fontana and colleagues[33] compared debridement with MACI in 30 patients with Tönnis grade 2 OA by radiographs, lesions greater than 2 cm^2, and Outerbridge grade 3 or 4 lesions. At 74 months, the debridement group HHS increased from 46 to 56.3. The MACI group increased from 48.3 to 87.4.[33] Fontana and de Girolamo[34] later reported 5-year results in 55 patients using autologous matrix-induced chondrogenesis, a similar single-stage technique whereby microfracture was performed underneath a collagen matrix that traps the progenitor cells within the defect. At all intervals except 1 year postoperatively, patients who underwent autologous matrix-induced chondrogenesis showed significant increase in their MHHS compared with a similar-sized group that underwent microfracture. Preoperatively, there was no difference in the mean size of the defects. Most subjects in both groups had lesions smaller than 4 cm^2. However, although the evidence suggests that MACI seems to have promise as a means to treat osteochondral defects of the hip, it is not currently approved for use in the United States.

Mosaicplasty

Mosaicplasty uses an array of cylindrical autologous osteochondral grafts to fill osteochondral defects. Autologous plugs are harvested from either the lateral trochlear ridge or the inferolateral femoral head. These plugs are then lightly inset into the field of the defect by debriding down to healthy base of surrounding cartilage and drilling recipient holes into the subchondral bone at the floor of the defect. The number of holes and therefore grafts depends on the size of the defect. **Fig. 3** shows the implantation of the graft into a femoral head defect. The procedure has been used with success in the knee for lesions up to 3 cm². Other indications include patients younger than 45 years of age with full-thickness defects and no OA.[35,36] In the hip, this has been used for osteochondral defects of the femoral head, particularly after trauma affecting the femur in a unipolar fashion. To date, there have been no reports of mosaicplasty being performed on the acetabular side. A significant benefit of mosaicplasty is the transplantation of hyaline tissue; this is a mechanical improvement compared with the fibrocartilage formed by microfracture. Nam and colleagues[37] showed incorporation of the grafts they performed in 2 patients who sustained femoral head lesions associated with posterior hip dislocation. Both patients returned to their baseline activity levels.[37] Hart and colleagues[38] reported a case in which the technique was used to treat a patient who sustained a femoral head lesion secondary to an acetabular fracture with concomitant posterior dislocation, and who subsequently failed the fixation. The patient had no pain and full hip range of motion, and the HHS improved from 69 to 100. Follow-up was more than 5 years.[38] Mosaicplasty has also been used in congenital and nontraumatic conditions affecting the femoral head cartilage. Sotereanos and colleagues[39] used the technique in a patient with AVN who had persistent pain in the hips after undergoing free fibular grafting. At the time of surgery, which was to be an arthroplasty, only a small area of femoral head cartilage was seen to be affected; total hip arthroplasty was abandoned and mosaicplasty performed. The patient's pain score significantly decreased.[39] It was performed in 10 patients with congenital hip conditions by Girard and colleagues,[40] on larger lesions than it would be indicated for in the knee, with an average size of nearly 5 cm². The HHS improved from 52.8 to 79.5 at an average of 29.2 months of follow-up. Computed tomography arthrograms were done at 6 months postoperatively, and showed excellent graft incorporation.[40] To facilitate mosaicplasty of the femoral head, a surgical dislocation is required. It has been done through a Smith-Peterson approach to further limit the risk of injury to the blood supply of the head. Emre and colleagues[41] reported a case of a femoral head defect in a 22-year-old that was dislocated in anterior fashion and treated with a 1.44-cm² graft from the ipsilateral knee. At 24 weeks postoperatively his HHS had gone from 43 to 96.[41] However, it does eliminate the need for a second-stage procedure such

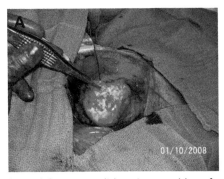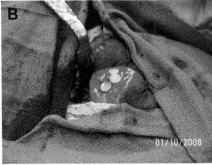

Fig. 3. (*A*) An open dislocation to address femoral head osteochondral disorder. This disorder was addressed with a mosaicplasty technique, the results of which are shown in (*B*). Care should be taken to inset the graft plugs just below the native chondral surface, and to attempt to orient them in a way that best matches the curvature of the femoral head; this helps limit abnormal contact pressures at the graft chondral surface.

as would be required with ACI. However, there is the risk of donor site morbidity, which has been reported to occur in ~3% of patients.[42]

Cartilage Repair

Microfracture relies on debriding the lesion of any unstable cartilage, down to subchondral surface. Meulenkamp and colleagues[43] showed that viable chondrocytes remain in the tissue removed in the process. Ten of the 12 cartilage flap samples obtained during their open treatment of FAI contained 50% or more hyaline cartilage. Only 2 specimens were predominantly fibrocartilage. This finding may provide the basis for successful attempts at repairing unstable but healthy delaminated cartilage, particularly in lesions more than 3 cm^2. As mentioned earlier, delaminated cartilage lesions are common sequelae of femoroacetabular impingement. Depending on the size of the lesion and its stability, the flap can either be treated as described with microfracture or, if larger than might be typically treated in this fashion, repair of the lesion using sutures or fibrin glue has been described.[44–46] Stafford and colleagues[44] used fibrin adhesive to treat 43 patients with delamination injuries, following them for an average of 28 months. MHHS in both the pain and function subscales were improved, from 21.8 to 35.8 and 40.0 to 43.6, respectively.[44] Other studies examining the results of cartilage repair have been on a smaller scale. Tzaveas and Villar[45] treated 19 patients' lesions with arthroscopic cartilage flap elevation, without resection, and microfracture. They then bonded the flap to the subchondral bone with fibrin glue. MHHS overall scores improved at 1 year's follow-up, as did the pain subscore, from 53.3 to 80.3 and 15.7 to 28.9, respectively. Twenty-six percent of their patients later underwent revision hip arthroscopy, in which the flap repairs were assessed and had remained stable in each.[45] A similar technique was used by Sekiya and colleagues,[46] who reported a case of unstable but healthy cartilage caused by FAI in a 17-year-old athlete. This 1-cm^2 lesion was sewn down rather than glued, using PDS suture after being elevated enough to facilitate microfracture. At 2 years, MHHS was 96. The Activities of Daily Living and Sports subscales of the Hip Outcome Score were 93 and 81, respectively.[46] Chondral lesions can also be associated with acute trauma, as in the case report of Lim and colleagues[47] describing femoral head disorder after an obturator dislocation.

Postoperative Care

During hip preservation several concomitant procedures may be performed and rehabilitation requires the surgeon to take all disorders into account. In general, the performance of a chondroplasty does not require postoperative restriction. The weight bearing of patients who undergo microfracture must be protected; the duration of this varies from 2 to 8 weeks before full weight bearing is allowed. Osteochondral transplantation, MACI/ACI, mosaicplasty, and articular cartilage repair are typically treated with 6 weeks of touch-down weight bearing and 6 weeks of partial weight bearing.

ALGORITHMS FOR TREATMENT

There are many options for surgical treatment. A simple algorithm has been proposed for managing these injuries.[6] This algorithm can be seen in **Fig. 4**, and can be used to aid in decision making when planning surgical interventions for the femur and acetabulum. As procedures become further refined and approved in the United States, it is likely that choosing among the various options will become more

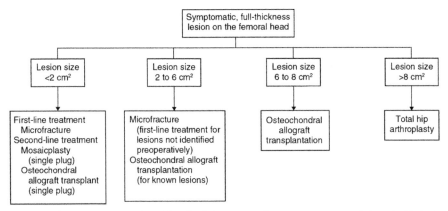

Fig. 4. Authors' treatment algorithm for joint-preserving management of chondral injuries of the femoral head. This algorithm can be used in patients who meet the following criteria: (1) age ranging from skeletal maturity to 50 years; (2) minimal (Tönnis grade ≤1) or no sign of osteoarthritis on radiography; (3) no inflammatory arthritis; (4) 1 or more full-thickness defects, but no bipolar lesions; (5) a well-contained lesion; (6) ability to perform rigorous postoperative physical therapy regimen.

complicated. At present, the treatment of osteochondral lesions of the hip fits well into this algorithm.

SUMMARY

Chondral injuries in young patients with hip disorders provide orthopedic surgeons with an opportunity to intervene early in the development of debilitating joint disease. Despite the challenges of managing these injuries, there are several reportedly successful options for treatment. Repair, microfracture, autograft chondrocytes, and allograft transplants have each been examined, albeit with small sample sizes and a paucity of head-to-head comparisons. However, the data continue to grow. As hip preservation matures, clearer recommendations for decision making regarding these treatments will emerge.

REFERENCES

1. McCarthy JC, Lee JA. Arthroscopic intervention in early hip disease. Clin Orthop Relat Res 2004;(429):157–62.
2. Domb BG, Redmond JM, Dunne KF, et al. A matched-pair controlled study of microfracture of the hip with average 2-year follow-up: do full-thickness chondral defects portend an inferior prognosis in hip arthroscopy? Arthroscopy 2015; 31(4):628–34.
3. Beck M, Leunig M, Parvizi J, et al. Anterior femoroacetabular impingement: part II. Midterm results of surgical treatment. Clin Orthop Relat Res 2004;(418):67–73.
4. Outerbridge RE. The etiology of chondromalacia patellae. J Bone Joint Surg Br 1961;43B:752–7.
5. Callaghan JJ, Rosenberg AG, Rubash HE. The adult hip. 2nd edition. Philadelphia: Lippincott Williams & Wilkins; 2007.
6. El Bitar YF, Lindner D, Jackson TJ, et al. Joint-preserving surgical options for management of chondral injuries of the hip. J Am Acad Orthop Surg 2014; 22(1):46–56.

7. Clohisy JC, Knaus ER, Hunt DM, et al. Clinical presentation of patients with symptomatic anterior hip impingement. Clin Orthop Relat Res 2009,407(3):638–44.

8. Beck M, Kalhor M, Leunig M, et al. Hip morphology influences the pattern of damage to the acetabular cartilage: femoroacetabular impingement as a cause of early osteoarthritis of the hip. J Bone Joint Surg Br 2005;87(7):1012–8.

9. Dooley PJ. Femoroacetabular impingement syndrome: Nonarthritic hip pain in young adults. Can Fam Physician 2008;54(1):42–7.

10. Ganz R, Parvizi J, Beck M, et al. Femoroacetabular impingement: a cause for osteoarthritis of the hip. Clin Orthop Relat Res 2003;(417):112–20.

11. Cunningham T, Jessel R, Zurakowski D, et al. Delayed gadolinium-enhanced magnetic resonance imaging of cartilage to predict early failure of Bernese periacetabular osteotomy for hip dysplasia. J Bone Joint Surg Am 2006;88(7): 1540–8.

12. Mont MA, Hungerford DS. Non-traumatic avascular necrosis of the femoral head. J Bone Joint Surg Am 1995;77(3):459–74.

13. Mont MA, Jones LC, Hungerford DS. Nontraumatic osteonecrosis of the femoral head: ten years later. J Bone Joint Surg Am 2006;88(5):1117–32.

14. Hirota Y, Hirohata T, Fukuda K, et al. Association of alcohol intake, cigarette smoking, and occupational status with the risk of idiopathic osteonecrosis of the femoral head. Am J Epidemiol 1993;137(5):530–8.

15. Yen YM, Kocher MS. Chondral lesions of the hip: microfracture and chondroplasty. Sports Med Arthrosc 2010;18(2):83–9.

16. Steadman JR, Briggs KK, Rodrigo JJ, et al. Outcomes of microfracture for traumatic chondral defects of the knee: average 11-year follow-up. Arthroscopy 2003;19(5):477–84.

17. Domb BG, Gupta A, Dunne KF, et al. Microfracture in the hip: results of a matched-cohort controlled study with 2-year follow-up. Am J Sports Med 2015; 43(8):1865–74.

18. Karthikeyan S, Roberts S, Griffin D. Microfracture for acetabular chondral defects in patients with femoroacetabular impingement: results at second-look arthroscopic surgery. Am J Sports Med 2012;40(12):2725–30.

19. Crawford K, Philippon MJ, Sekiya JK, et al. Microfracture of the hip in athletes. Clin Sports Med 2006;25(2):327–35, x.

20. Haughom BD, Erickson BJ, Rybalko D, et al. Arthroscopic acetabular microfracture with the use of flexible drills: a technique guide. Arthrosc Tech 2014;3(4): e459–63.

21. Frisbie DD, Oxford JT, Southwood L, et al. Early events in cartilage repair after subchondral bone microfracture. Clin Orthop Relat Res 2003;(407):215–27.

22. Philippon MJ, Schenker ML, Briggs KK, et al. Can microfracture produce repair tissue in acetabular chondral defects? Arthroscopy 2008;24(1):46–50.

23. Byrd JW, Jones KS. Osteoarthritis caused by an inverted acetabular labrum: radiographic diagnosis and arthroscopic treatment. Arthroscopy 2002;18(7): 741–7.

24. Byrd JW, Jones KS. Arthroscopic femoroplasty in the management of cam-type femoroacetabular impingement. Clin Orthop Relat Res 2009;467(3):739–46.

25. Horisberger M, Brunner A, Herzog RF. Arthroscopic treatment of femoral acetabular impingement in patients with preoperative generalized degenerative changes. Arthroscopy 2010;26(5):623–9.

26. Philippon MJ, Briggs KK, Yen YM, et al. Outcomes following hip arthroscopy for femoroacetabular impingement with associated chondrolabral dysfunction: minimum two-year follow-up. J Bone Joint Surg Br 2009;91(1):16–23.

27. Krych AJ, Lorich DG, Kelly BT. Treatment of focal osteochondral defects of the acetabulum with osteochondral allograft transplantation. Orthopedics 2011; 34(7):e307–11.

28. Williams RJ 3rd, Ranawat AS, Potter HG, et al. Fresh stored allografts for the treatment of osteochondral defects of the knee. J Bone Joint Surg Am 2007;89(4): 718–26.

29. Meyers MH. Resurfacing of the femoral head with fresh osteochondral allografts. Long-term results. Clin Orthop Relat Res 1985;(197):111–4.

30. Ganz R, Gill TJ, Gautier E, et al. Surgical dislocation of the adult hip a technique with full access to the femoral head and acetabulum without the risk of avascular necrosis. J Bone Joint Surg Br 2001;83(8):1119–24.

31. Fontana A. A novel technique for treating cartilage defects in the hip: a fully arthroscopic approach to using autologous matrix-induced chondrogenesis. Arthrosc Tech 2012;1(1):e63–8.

32. Akimau P, Bhosale A, Harrison PE, et al. Autologous chondrocyte implantation with bone grafting for osteochondral defect due to posttraumatic osteonecrosis of the hip–a case report. Acta Orthop 2006;77(2):333–6.

33. Fontana A, Bistolfi A, Crova M, et al. Arthroscopic treatment of hip chondral defects: autologous chondrocyte transplantation versus simple debridement–a pilot study. Arthroscopy 2012;28(3):322–9.

34. Fontana A, de Girolamo L. Sustained five-year benefit of autologous matrix-induced chondrogenesis for femoral acetabular impingement-induced chondral lesions compared with microfracture treatment. Bone Joint J 2015;97B(5): 628–35.

35. Gudas R, Gudaite A, Pocius A, et al. Ten-year follow-up of a prospective, randomized clinical study of mosaic osteochondral autologous transplantation versus microfracture for the treatment of osteochondral defects in the knee joint of athletes. Am J Sports Med 2012;40(11):2499–508.

36. Marcacci M, Kon E, Delcogliano M, et al. Arthroscopic autologous osteochondral grafting for cartilage defects of the knee: prospective study results at a minimum 7-year follow-up. Am J Sports Med 2007;35(12).2014–21.

37. Nam D, Shindle MK, Buly RL, et al. Traumatic osteochondral injury of the femoral head treated by mosaicplasty: a report of two cases. Hss J 2010;6(2):228–34.

38. Hart R, Janecek M, Visna P, et al. Mosaicplasty for the treatment of femoral head defect after incorrect resorbable screw insertion. Arthroscopy 2003;19(10):E1–5.

39. Sotereanos NG, DeMeo PJ, Hughes TB, et al. Autogenous osteochondral transfer in the femoral head after osteonecrosis. Orthopedics 2008;31(2):177.

40. Girard J, Roumazeille T, Sakr M, et al. Osteochondral mosaicplasty of the femoral head. Hip Int 2011;21(5):542–8.

41. Emre TY, Cift H, Seyhan B, et al. Mosaicplasty for the treatment of the osteochondral lesion in the femoral head. Bull NYU Hosp Jt Dis 2012;70(4):288–90.

42. Hangody L, Rathonyi GK, Duska Z, et al. Autologous osteochondral mosaicplasty. Surgical technique. J Bone Joint Surg Am 2004;86A(Suppl 1):65–72.

43. Meulenkamp B, Gravel D, Beaule PE. Viability assessment of the chondral flap in patients with cam-type femoroacetabular impingement: a preliminary report. Can J Surg 2014;57(1):44–8.

44. Stafford GH, Bunn JR, Villar RN. Arthroscopic repair of delaminated acetabular articular cartilage using fibrin adhesive. Results at one to three years. Hip Int 2011;21(6):744–50.

45. Tzaveas AP, Villar RN. Arthroscopic repair of acetabular chondral delamination with fibrin adhesive. Hip Int 2010;20(1):115–9.

46. Sekiya JK, Martin RL, Lesniak BP. Arthroscopic repair of delaminated acetabular articular cartilage in femoroacetabular impingement. Orthopedics 2009;32(9).
47. Lim BH, Jang SW, Park YS, et al. Open repair and arthroscopic follow-up of severely delaminated femoral head cartilage associated with traumatic obturator fracture-dislocation of the hip. Orthopedics 2011;34(6):199.

Capsular Management in Hip Arthroscopy

Joshua D. Harris, MD[a,b]

KEYWORDS

- Iliofemoral ligament • Hip capsule • Capsulotomy • Capsular repair
- Capsular plication • Capsular reconstruction • Zona orbicularis • Microinstability

KEY POINTS

- The iliofemoral ligament is the strongest component of the hip capsule but is divided (perpendicular) with the interportal capsulotomy.
- Capsular repair (of either the interportal or T capsulotomy) restores rotational and translational biomechanics of the hip joint.
- Greater degrees of plication may be titrated in patients with risk factors for postoperative instability (Ehlers-Danlos, connective tissue disorders, ballet dancers, gymnastics, yoga).
- Sufficient capsular incision is necessary to achieve the osseous (impingement) and soft tissue (chondrolabral) goals of the arthroscopic hip preservation procedure.

INTRODUCTION

Arthroscopic hip preservation is one of the most rapidly growing and evolving fields in orthopedic surgery. Variable degrees of capsular incision are required for joint access, visualization, and instrumentation. Controversy exists regarding the type, size, and location of capsulotomy necessary to properly address central and peripheral compartment pathology. Controversy does not exist regarding the necessity to correct symptomatic femoroacetabular impingement (FAI) osseous morphology. The surgeon must be able to visualize the morphology in order to treat it. Closure, plication, shift, and reconstruction are a few options available to address the capsulotomy at the conclusion of the surgery. However, this component of capsular management is technically challenging and requires meticulous technique for optimal outcomes.

Source of Funding: None.

Disclosures: Editorial board: *Arthroscopy: The Journal of Arthroscopic and Related Surgery; Frontiers In Surgery*; research support: Smith and Nephew, Depuy Synthes; publication royalties: SLACK, Inc; committees: AOSSM Self-Assessment Committee, AAOS Osteoarthritis Pain and Function Workgroup.

[a] Department of Orthopedics & Sports Medicine, Houston Methodist Hospital Institute for Academic Medicine, 6550 Fannin Street, Smith Tower, Suite 2500, Houston, TX 77030, USA;
[b] Weill Cornell Medical College, New York, NY 10065, USA
E-mail address: joshuaharrismd@gmail.com

NORMAL CAPSULE ANATOMY

The hip is a deep, constrained, diarthrodial synovial joint, surrounded by a thick musculotendinous soft tissue envelope. Although the capsule seems to dichotomize hip anatomy into 2 compartments, intra-articular and extra-articular, the layer concept of hip anatomy describes a method to determine the sources of hip pathology and subsequent treatment.[1] The osteochondral layer, layer I, provides the basis for arthrokinetic motion via joint congruity. Hip motion is primarily rotational, around a center of rotation, rather than translational.[2] Within layer I, loss of head-neck junction sphericity (cam FAI), femoral head overcoverage (pincer FAI) or undercoverage (dysplasia), and extra-articular impingement (anterior inferior iliac spine [AIIS] subspine impingement, trochanteric-pelvic, ischiofemoral) may all disrupt normal joint mechanics (translation in addition to rotation). Other osseous femoral (version, neck-shaft angle), acetabular (version, depth), and lumbopelvic (pelvic incidence, sagittal and coronal plane balance) parameters play a significant role in evaluation of layer I anatomy and pathology.

Layer II is composed of the inert, noncontractile soft tissue structures in and around the hip, including the labrum and the capsule. Although the fibrocartilaginous labrum provides a joint-stabilizing suction seal during motion, the capsule provides a joint-stabilizing check-rein to both translational and rotational ends of range of motion. Both structures resist femoral head axial distraction out of the acetabulum. The capsule is composed of 4 discrete ligamentous structures: iliofemoral (anterior), ischiofemoral (posterior), pubofemoral (inferior), and zona orbicularis (circumferential at head-neck junction). The iliofemoral ligament is the strongest of the 4 and is transversely cut during interportal capsulotomy (anterolateral [AL] to midanterior) in hip arthroscopy.[3] The latter permits excellent viewing of the central compartment: labrum, acetabular rim, articular cartilage of the acetabulum and femoral head, fovea, and ligamentum teres. A T capsulotomy, perpendicular to the interportal capsulotomy, permits excellent viewing of the peripheral compartment: proximal femoral head-neck junction, zona orbicularis, lateral and medial synovial folds, and lateral ascending vessels. Several biomechanical investigations have illustrated the importance of the iliofemoral ligament for retention of normal hip kinematics: Iliofemoral ligament sectioning (unrepaired capsulotomy) leads to increased external rotation, extension, and anterior and distal translation (**Table 1**).[4–9] An unrepaired T capsulotomy may potentially leave the hip catastrophically unstable (dislocation) or prone to microinstability due to a disrupted "stability arc."[10] The "stability arc" is a defined area of the anterior hip, defined by the medial and lateral limbs of the iliofemoral ligament as the static deep border and the iliocapsularis and rectus femoris as the dynamic superficial medial border and the gluteus minimus as the dynamic superficial lateral border (**Fig. 1**A).[10] In the setting of an unrepaired T capsulotomy, hip extension and external rotation dynamically pull the medial and lateral limbs of the iliofemoral ligament apart and evade the anterior stabilizing effect of the anterior capsule due to the pull of the iliocapsularis and gluteus minimus (layer III structures), respectively (see **Fig. 1**B). Layer III consists of the dynamic musculotendinous units in and around the hip and pelvis. This layer includes the muscles whose action is to move the hip, the lumbopelvic stabilizing girdle, and the pelvic floor. Layer IV is composed of the neurokinetic layer, the thoraco-lumbo-sacral plexus, and lumbopelvic tissues, serving as the neural link to the hip and lower extremities.

CAPSULAR PATHOPHYSIOLOGY

There are 2 settings in which capsular deficiency may exist: iatrogenic and native. Iatrogenic capsular insufficiency may exist in patients having undergone hip arthroscopy with an unrepaired capsulotomy (**Fig. 2**).[11] As the interportal capsulotomy directly incises the iliofemoral ligament perpendicular to the line of its fibers, if left

Table 1		
Role of hip capsule in instability		
Study	**Study Design**	**Role**
Jackson et al,[4] 2015	Cadaveric biomechanical: motion tracking	• Vented, instability (increased extension; increased ER, distraction), interportal capsulotomy, repair, shift models • Instability model = 35 Nm extension torque applied to intact hip in neutral rotation • Instability state increased extension (9.3° to 16.0°; $P = .009$); ER (26° to 31°; $P = .045$), IR (from 5° extension to 45° flexion; $P<.05$ for all) • Interportal capsulotomy increased IR, ER, extension, distraction ($P<.05$ for all) • Capsular repair restored IR to instability, but not intact, state, at 0° and 5° extension; restored ER at all degrees ROM, restored distraction to instability, but not intact state; restored extension to intact • Capsular shift decreased IR (overtightened) from 5° extension to 15° flexion; restored ER, distraction, and extension to intact state
Abrams et al,[5] 2015	Cadaveric biomechanical: motion tracking	• 0°, 40° testing states for intact, interportal, T capsulotomy, complete capsular repair, capsulectomy • Increase ER with T capsulotomy ($P = .03$) and capsulectomy ($P = .02$); no difference in ER after T repair • No difference in ER between groups at 40° flexion • No difference in ER between intact and interportal capsulotomy at 0° flexion
Bayne et al,[6] 2014	Cadaveric biomechanical: motion tracking	• Interportal capsulotomy: increased distal, lateral, and anterior translation in neutral (more translation than rotation) • Interportal capsulotomy: increased distal, medial, and posterior translation in flexion (more rotation than translation)
Myers et al,[8] 2011	Cadaveric biomechanical: fluoroscopy	• Increased external rotation with IFL sectioning (increased 12.9°) ($P<.0001$) • Increased anterior translation with IFL sectioning (increased 1.8 mm) ($P<.001$) • No difference in external rotation or anterior translation between intact/repaired state
Martin et al,[7] 2008	Cadaveric biomechanical: motion tracking	• Release of medial, lateral arms IFL gave greatest increase of external rotation • Lateral arm release provides more motion in flexion and neutral • Lateral arm release also provides more internal rotation, primarily in extension
Hewitt et al,[9] 2002	Cadaveric biomechanical: load to failure	• IFL much stronger than the ischiofemoral ligaments • IFL greater stiffness than ischiofemoral ligaments • IFL greater tensile load to failure than ischiofemoral ligaments

Abbreviations: ER, external rotation; IFL, iliofemoral ligament; IR, internal rotation; ROM, range of motion.

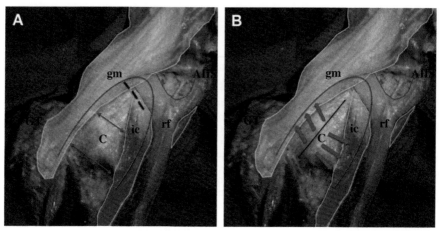

Fig. 1. (*A*) Anterior view of right hip illustrating stability arc borders (*red solid line*). The 2 red lines with arrows illustrate the persistent dynamic tensioning that occurs across the intact anterior capsule as the 2 limbs of the arc contract to stabilize the hip in extension and external rotation. The dashed black line illustrates the location of the interportal capsulotomy. (*B*) Anterior view of right hip illustrating stability arc borders (*red solid line*). The solid black line illustrates the location of the *T* capsulotomy. The red lines with arrows show how an unrepaired capsulotomy leads to persistent dynamic tensioning of the capsular flaps away from one another as their respective muscles contract during extension and external rotation. C, capsule; gm, gluteus minimus; GT, greater trochanter; ic, iliocapsularis; rf, rectus femoris. (*From* Walters BL, Cooper JH, Rodriguez JA. New findings in hip capsular anatomy: dimensions of capsular thickness and pericapsular contributions. Arthroscopy 2014;30(10):1235–45; with permission.)

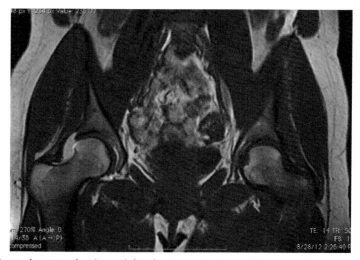

Fig. 2. Coronal proton density-weighted anteroposterior pelvis magnetic resonance arthrogram in a 22-year-old woman 1 year after right hip arthroscopy and an unrepaired interportal capsulotomy.

unrepaired, the femoral head may demonstrate both abnormal rotation[4–9] and translation.[4,6] The *T* capsulotomy may further destabilize the hip if left unrepaired.[4,5] If left unrepaired, 2 scenarios may occur: (1) microinstability (defined as femoral head translation, in addition to rotation)[12,13] and (2) macroinstability (defined as femoral head subluxation or dislocation).[14] In the laboratory, complete capsular repair of interportal and *T* capsulotomies has been shown to normalize both rotation and translation.[3,5] Native capsular insufficiency may exist in patients with multiple various connective tissue disorders, Ehlers-Danlos, Beighton score greater than 4, hypermobility joint syndrome, ballet dancers, gymnasts, figure skaters, or mixed martial arts. Further, in patients with FAI, using 3-dimensional (3D) computed tomography (CT), anterior impingement demonstrated posterior subluxation in 70% of patients, whereas posterior impingement demonstrated anterior subluxation in 40% of patients.[15]

INDICATIONS

The indications for capsular repair have undergone a significant evolution over time with improved understanding of the importance of capsular anatomy, improved instrumentation, and improved surgical technique. At the conclusion of the arthroscopy and before capsular closure begins the most technically demanding portion of the surgery. Although unrepaired capsulotomies and/or capsulectomies have been used as therapeutic interventions in the past, these are typically in stiff, osteoarthritic patients. These interventions have been performed either open or arthroscopically. Given that hip arthroscopy is generally not indicated as a treatment in patients with osteoarthritis, leaving a capsule unrepaired or removed is never indicated in nonarthritic patients (**Box 1**).

CONTRAINDICATIONS

There are 2 absolute contraindications to capsular repair in patients undergoing arthroscopic hip preservation, and they are relegated to the contraindication to arthroscopy rather than the repair itself. A capsular repair or plication cannot be used to stabilize a hip with significant dysplasia (more than borderline or mild dysplasia: break in the Shenton line, femoral head extrusion index >25%, lateral center edge angle less than 20°, anterior center edge angle less than 20°, and Tonnis angle >15°).[16] The same concept applies to patients with significant osteoarthritis: Tonnis grade 2 or 3 or in patients with less than 2 mm of joint space.[17]

Box 1
Indications and contraindications for capsular repair in hip arthroscopy

Indications

- Hip arthroscopy in patients with soft tissue risk factors for postoperative instability
  - Ehlers-Danlos
  - Connective tissue disorder
  - Beighton score greater than 4
  - Benign joint hypermobility syndrome
  - Flexibility sport athlete (eg, ballet, gymnastics)
- Hip arthroscopy in nonarthritic patients
- Hip arthroscopy in nondysplastic and borderline dysplastic patients

Contraindications

- Hip arthroscopy in patients with moderate or severe dysplasia
- Hip arthroscopy in patients with hip osteoarthritis

SURGICAL TECHNIQUE
Preoperative Planning

Meticulous consideration of patients' subjective and objective evaluation, including chief complaint, history of present illness, and physical examination, must be carefully corroborated with patients' imaging investigations (plain radiographs, MRI, CT) ("treat the patient, not the MRI").

Patient Positioning

Patients are positioned on the table to optimize arthroscopic access to the hip joint. Although the author prefers the supine position, lateral decubitus is also a viable option. General anesthesia with complete muscle relaxation assists in reduction of force necessary to obtain sufficient distraction (less than 50–100 lb) for atraumatic entry into the joint.[18,19] A well-padded perineal post (minimum of 9 cm) and a greater lateral vector of distraction are associated with reduced pressure on the pudendal nerve (perineal and dorsal genital branches).[18,19] In fact, for every 1-lb increase in distraction force applied, there is a 4% odds increase of an adverse nerve event (lateral position arthroscopy).[19] Although the amount of time in traction has not been shown to influence the risk of a postoperative nerve event in either supine or lateral positions, the duration of time should be kept to less than 2 hours to reduce the risk of compressive, ischemic tourniquetlike injury to the nerves in the perineum.[19,20] In order to circumvent the risk of perineal injury, some investigators have successfully performed hip arthroscopy without a post without a single documented groin or perineum complication.[21,22] The most common complication of hip arthroscopy is iatrogenic articular cartilage or labral injury (0.4% to 3.8% and 0.7% to 18.0%, respectively), which occurs primarily with portal placement.[23–28] Thus, patient positioning must optimize the ability to successfully place portals. Several investigations have reported technical pearls for reducing, and even potentially eliminating, the risk of iatrogenic injury.[28–31] The learning curve for hip arthroscopy has been shown to range from 20 to more than 100 cases, with a reduction in the incidence of iatrogenic chondrolabral injury with greater surgeon experience.[26,32–34]

Surgical Procedure

1. The patient's appropriate hip is selected and marked in the preoperative holding area after verbal and written informed consent. The patient is taken to the operating theater and general anesthesia is induced; complete muscle paralysis is obtained; parenteral antibiotics are administered (no more than 30 minutes before skin incision: cefazolin 1 g intravenous [2 g if patient is 75 kg body weight or greater]; clindamycin 600 mg intravenous if allergic to cephalosporin allergy).

2. Examination under anesthesia is performed. This examination includes measurement of bilateral hip flexion, abduction, and internal and external rotation at 90° hip flexion. Assessment of external rotation recoil, dial testing (maximal limb internal rotation and permissive passive external rotation assessment for end point and >45° of external rotation), and traction testing (with or without fluoroscopic assistance) all evaluate capsular (especially the iliofemoral ligament) integrity. Fluoroscopic examination under anesthesia can be helpful to accurately identify trochanteric-pelvic and ischiofemoral impingement. Femoral head translation, in addition to rotation, may also be fluoroscopically observed if the head-neck junction levers on the acetabular fulcrum (microinstability) with or without the presence of a vacuum sign.[12,13,16]

3. A surgical pause time-out is performed before operative limb distraction is commenced. The patient is slid down the operative table (Advanced Supine Hip

Positioning System with 2 Universal Hip Distractors and 2 Active Heel Traction Boots; Smith & Nephew, Andover, MA) with a well-padded perineal post between the legs. The post is eccentrically placed toward the operative side, to increase the lateral vector during distraction and reduce the pressure on the perineum. Each boot should be placed and Velcro strapped so that no creases, rivets, or grooves indent the patient's foot or ankle. A self-adherent elastic cohesive bandage is applied over the boot to increase the coefficients of friction in the Active Heel Traction Boot to reduce the risk of the foot pulling out of the boot.

4. The nonoperative limb is placed in 5° flexion, 45° abduction, and neutral rotation. A gentle longitudinal axial distractive force is applied to simply take any slack out of the limb and provide a countertraction lateral vector force to the operative side. The operative limb is placed in approximately 30° abduction and 30° of flexion in neutral rotation. Slow gentle adduction is applied to approximately 0° abduction, then in a slow, gentle application of zigzagging hip extension-adduction, extension-adduction, extension-adduction moments, the operative limb is placed in approximately 5° flexion, 5° adduction, and neutral rotation. The limb is then internally rotated to the degree of femoral anteversion (measured from preoperative CT scan) (if 15° anteversion, then 15° internal rotation). The C-arm fluoroscopic unit is able to be placed between the legs and not interfere with the surgeon or limb manipulation before or after traction application.

5. Sterile preparation and draping of the limb with an Isolation Drape with Incise Film and Pouch (3M Health Care, St Paul, MN) allows for quick and easy application of a surgical drape that protects the sterile field and covers the patient's body. Using a sterile marker, a straight line is drawn connecting the anterior superior iliac spine and the patella. No portal should be established at or medial to this line.

6. Portal placement is one of the most critical aspects of the procedure, establishing the access for visualization and instrumentation of the joint. The AL portal is established first, using a 17-gauge spinal needle, aimed to enter the joint at the 12:30 position on the acetabular clock face (in a right hip). Fluoroscopy is used to assist in AL portal placement. The Seldinger technique is used to place a 4.5-mm cannula and introduce the 70° arthroscope. The anterior triangle is visualized; using spinal needle localization, a modified midanterior portal (MMAP) is created, entering the joint at the 3:00 position on the clock face (**Fig. 3**A). On the surface, this is approximately 4 to 6 cm medial and 2 to 4 cm distal to the AL portal.

7. Proper capsular management begins with portal placement and creation of the capsulotomy. An interportal capsulotomy is created using an arthroscopic 4.0-mm Beaver Blade (Smith & Nephew; Andover, MA). The capsulotomy should be sharp, avoiding fraying of the perpendicular cut in the fibers of the iliofemoral ligament. The incision should be approximately 5 to 8 mm away from the labrum. The further distal from the labrum, the greater amount of tissue available for repair at case conclusion. The author does not typically extend the capsulotomy beyond 3:00, as this opens the potential for fluid extravasation up the iliopsoas tendon sheath to the pelvis and abdomen. Depending on patient size, the length of the capsulotomy is variably 2 to 4 cm in length. Posterior to 12:00, the capsule becomes thin and largely deficient, blending into the ischiofemoral ligament. From portal placement to interportal capsulotomy creation, the author prefers dry arthroscopy before fluid is introduced and the potential for a redout is reduced. The lateral component of the capsulotomy is made while viewing from the MMAP portal (see **Fig. 3**B). The medial component of the capsulotomy is made while viewing from the AL portal (see **Fig. 3**C). Minimizing the amount of capsulectomy helps for capsular repair at the end of the case. Although capsular

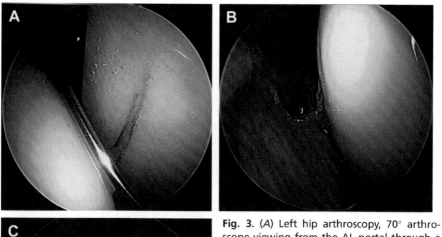

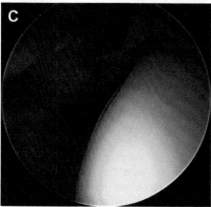

Fig. 3. (A) Left hip arthroscopy, 70° arthroscope viewing from the AL portal through a 4.5-mm cannula, viewing the anterior triangle. A 17-gauge spinal has been placed at approximately the 3:00 position and a nitinol wire used via Seldinger technique for placement of a 5.0-mm cannula in the MMAP. (B) A 70° arthroscope viewing from MMAP back toward AL portal while creating lateral portion of interportal capsulotomy with Beaver Blade. (C) Right hip arthroscopy, 70° arthroscope viewing from AL portal while creating medial portion of interportal capsulotomy with Beaver Blade. (Courtesy of Joshua D. Harris, MD.)

debridement does improve visualization, it makes capsular repair more challenging and may overconstrain the anterior hip because of the amount of plication.[4]

8. Central compartment diagnostic arthroscopy
   a. Labrum, chondrolabral junction
   b. Articular cartilage: femoral head, acetabulum
   c. Fovea, ligamentum teres
   d. Acetabular rim
   e. AIIS

9. To assist with evaluation of the acetabular rim without capsulectomy, traction sutures placed in each limb of the capsule help lift the capsule off the rim, visualize the capsulolabral interval, and treat acetabular-sided pathology (pincer and subspine impingement).[35,36] Labral repair may be performed with either 2 portals (MMAP, AL) or with 3 (MMAP, AL, and distal anterolateral accessory [DALA] portal). The DALA portal is created with spinal needle localization, entering the skin approximately 4 cm distal to the AL portal.

10. Once central compartment arthroscopy concludes, traction is discontinued. During peripheral compartment arthroscopy, an assistant may manipulate the limb with variable combinations of flexion, abduction, and rotation. The author typically uses 6 anteroposterior fluoroscopic views (3 views in hip extension [30° external

rotation, 30° internal rotation, neutral] and 3 views in 50° flexion [neutral, 40° external rotation, 60° external rotation]) that correlate with preoperative 3D CT scan to help visualize and correct the typical cam morphology from 11:45 to 2:45. Although the use of traction sutures does assist in peripheral compartment visualization with MMAP and AL portals, the author prefers to create a *T* capsulotomy.

11. The precapsular fat pad is gently debrided with a mechanical shaver to expose the interval between the iliocapsularis (medial) and gluteus minimus (lateral). This intermuscular plane exposes the location for the *T* capsulotomy, which is created using a 3.0-mm radiofrequency probe (Dyonics RF Hook 30° Probe; Smith & Nephew, Andover, MA) down the anterolateral femoral neck to the intertrochanteric line (**Fig. 4**). The *T* begins at the midpoint between the medial and lateral ends of the interportal capsulotomy. As with the interportal capsulotomy, minimal to no capsulectomy should be performed. Traction sutures may be placed in each limb of the *T* for complete visualization of more than 180° of the head-neck junction, the lateral ascending vessels, and the medial and lateral synovial folds. While visualizing from the MMAP, the author uses a SpeedStitch device (ArthroCare Sports Medicine, Austin, TX) through the AL portal to place one traction suture in the lateral limb and through the DALA portal to place one traction suture in the medial limb of the *T* capsulotomy.

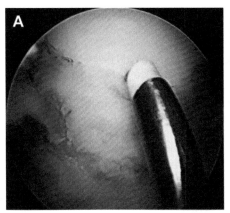
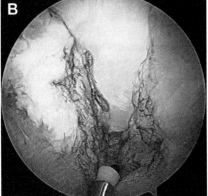
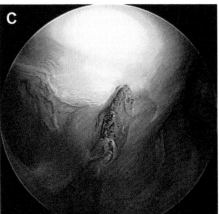

Fig. 4. Right hip arthroscopy, 70° arthroscope viewing from MMAP, while beginning the T capsulotomy using a Dyonics RF Hook 30° Probe (*A*); extending distally anterolateral down the femoral neck toward the intertrochanteric line (*B*); and the approximately 180° of femoral head-neck junction exposure after traction sutures placed in both limbs of the *T* capsulotomy (*C*). (*Courtesy of* Joshua D. Harris, MD.)

12. Cam osteoplasty is performed using the knowledge of preoperative imaging, intraoperative landmarks (hard, sclerotic cortical bone), and fluoroscopic views for a complete correction.

13. All bony debris is evacuated at the conclusion of the osteoplasty.

14. *T* closure commences with placement of an 8.5-mm cannula in the DALA portal. Multiple capsular closure devices may be used. Given the technical difficulty associated with capsular repair, the author recommends using multiple devices in the laboratory setting, finding the one most reproducible in the surgeon's hands, and learning adaptability of different devices for different patients. Greater degrees of plication or capsular shift may require larger bites of tissue that only certain devices can achieve.

15. The most distal aspect of the *T* is closed first, and the closure proceeds proximal toward the interportal capsulotomy (**Fig. 5A–E**). On average, 3 high-strength nonabsorbable No. 2 sutures are used in the *T* (see **Fig. 5F**). A side-to-side closure is usually performed with no shift desired. In patients with risk factors for hip microinstability (Ehlers-Danlos, connective tissue disorders, Beighton score >4, hypermobility joint syndrome, ballet dancers, gymnasts, figure skaters, mixed martial arts, borderline dysplasia), the author uses a 70° up SlingShot (Pivot Medical, Sunnyvale, CA) to perform a capsular plication. The SlingShot secures approximately 2 cm of suture in its penetrating needle and retriever. The surgeon then passes the needle and suture through the medial limb with an approximately 5- to 8-mm bite of tissue. The suture is deployed deep to the capsule and the needle removed and then repositioned over the lateral limb. The needle then pierces and retrieves the suture through the lateral limb at an approximately 5- to 8-mm bite of lateral tissue. The greater the potential of instability, the greater the plication performed. The author ties each suture, using reversing half hitches on alternating posts, sequentially, rather than passing all 3 sutures and then tying. In patients without any risk factors for instability, the author uses a SpeedStitch, placing 5 mm or less bites of tissue on each limb of the *T*. Using the SpeedStitch, the author typically passes 3 sutures to close the *T*.

16. The arthroscope is then placed in AL portal and the 8.5-mm cannula placed in the MMAP. In patients with instability risk factors, the SlingShot is used. An inferior capsular shift may be performed for an even greater amount of iliofemoral ligament plication.[37] The distal (femoral) side of the interportal capsulotomy is pierced with suture first, further medial than the more lateral location of the proximal (acetabular) side of the capsulotomy (**Fig. 6A**). Approximately 5-mm bites are grasped on both sides of the capsulotomy (see **Fig. 6B**). Usually 3 sutures are used for interportal closure, with 2 medial to the *T* and one lateral to the *T*. All 3 sutures are passed first and then tied from medial to lateral. The hip is held in 0° flexion during interportal closure to avoid overtightening. Complete capsular closure is verified when articular cartilage, labrum, and neck osteoplasty are no longer visible (see **Fig. 6C**).

17. Portal closure is performed using a 3-0 nonabsorbable polypropylene (Prolene) suture. Sterile dressing is applied.

POSTOPERATIVE CARE

1. A hinged hip brace is applied in the operating room and fitted to the patient preoperatively. This brace limits hip extension: no flexion beyond 90° and no abduction. The brace is used for 4 weeks following surgery.

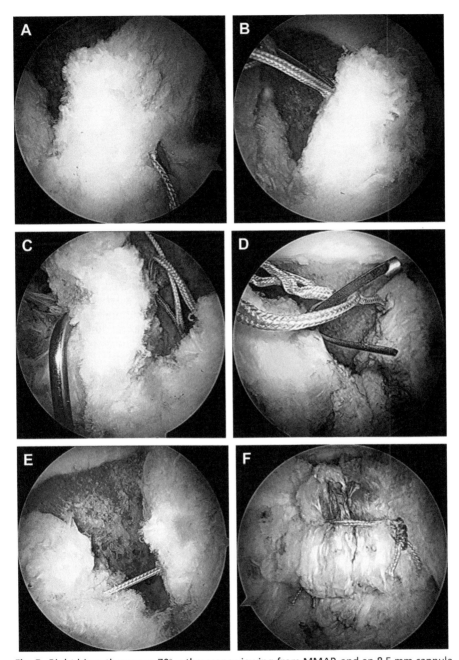

Fig. 5. Right hip arthroscopy, 70° arthroscope viewing from MMAP, and an 8.5-mm cannula placed in the DALA. A 70° SlingShot is used to pierce the medial limb (*A*); push the high-strength nonabsorbable No. 2 suture through the device (*B*); then, without removing the device from the cannula, piercing the lateral limb (*C*); retrieving the suture (*D*); and preparing to tie arthroscopic knots (reversing half hitches on alternating posts) (*E*). The author ties each knot sequentially for each suture, rather than passing all sutures and tying last. Completed *T* limb closure with 3 sutures (*F*). (*Courtesy of* Joshua D. Harris, MD.)

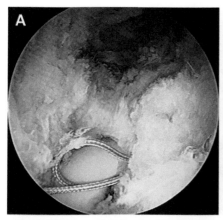

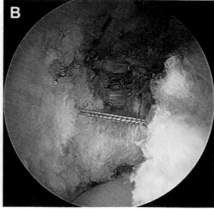

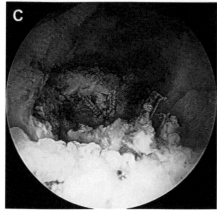

Fig. 6. Right hip arthroscopy, 70° arthroscope viewing from AL portal, and an 8.5-mm cannula placed in the MMAP. A 70° SlingShot is used to pierce the distal limb first (*A*); further medial than where grabbed through the proximal limb (in effect, generating an inferior capsular shift) (*B*); 3 sutures are typically used; in a complete closure, no femoral head is visible (*C*). (*Courtesy of* Joshua D. Harris, MD.)

2. Derotational boots are used for 2 to 3 weeks following surgery while sleeping to prevent the extended and externally rotated position that will stress the capsular closure.
3. Crutch-assisted, foot-flat partial (20 lb) weight bearing is used for 4 to 6 weeks following surgery.
4. Formal physical therapy commences on postoperative day one, with gentle passive motion, circumduction exercises, limited rotational stress, and avoidance of iliopsoas activation and overutilization.
5. Standard oral pain medications are used, in addition to stool softeners (if narcotics), heterotopic ossification prophylaxis (4 days of 75 mg oral indomethacin, followed by 4 weeks of 500 mg oral naproxen twice daily), esomeprazole (20 mg oral, once daily) for 4 weeks and 4 days, and 325 mg aspirin twice daily for chemical thromboembolic disease prophylaxis for 3 weeks.

COMPLICATIONS AND MANAGEMENT

The complications related to capsular management are typically due to unrepaired capsulotomies, which may introduce the potential for postoperative instability: microinstability or macroinstability. In the 11 cases of hip dislocation or subluxation following hip arthroscopy, only one used a *T* capsulotomy, which was not repaired.[14,38–47] In the 10 macroinstability cases, variable sizes of interportal capsulotomies were created. However, only 2 were repaired. Although hip dislocation following arthroscopy is likely highly multifactorial, the unrepaired capsulotomy plays a clear role. For nonarthritic, nondysplastic patients with symptomatic microinstability following primary hip arthroscopy that required revision arthroscopy (n = 33), Wylie and colleagues[48] demonstrated significantly ($P<.05$ for all) improved modified Harris Hip Scores and Hip Outcome Scores (activities of daily and sports subscales) at a 2-year minimum follow-up.

OUTCOMES

Clinical outcome studies are limited with respect to the capsular contribution to outcome (**Table 2**). Frank and colleagues[49] demonstrated a significantly better outcome with complete capsular repair of a *T* capsulotomy versus a partial repair at the 6-, 12-, and 30-month follow-up. The partial repair group had a 13% revision rate for instability, whereas the complete repair group required no revisions. Larson and colleagues[50] performed primary FAI correction in an extreme soft tissue laxity situation in 16 patients with Ehlers-Danlos syndrome at the 44-month follow-up. Patients demonstrated significant improvements ($P<.05$) in Short Form-12 (SF-12), visual analog scale pain score, and modified Harris Hip Score ($\Delta43$ points from before to after surgery). In a separate investigation of revision FAI correction, Larson and colleagues[51] examined the influence of capsular plication and showed a significant ($P = .032$) influence on better-modified Harris Hip Score at the 26-month follow-up in patients undergoing capsular plication.

Table 2
Arthroscopic hip preservation outcome with respect to capsule

Authors	Number of Subjects	Cohorts	Outcome
Wylie et al,[38] 2015	33	33 Hips symptomatic instability after primary arthroscopy	• Significant improvements in modified Harris Hip Score and Hip Outcome Score subscores at minimum 1- and 2-year follow-up
Larson et al,[50] 2015	16	Ehlers-Danlos and FAI undergoing FAI correction and capsular plication	• At 3.5-year follow-up, significantly improved modified Harris Hip Score, visual analog pain score, and SF-12 score • One revision capsular plication
Frank et al,[49] 2014	64	32 Subjects complete repair; 32 subjects partial repair	• Significantly better outcome in complete repair group in Hip Outcome Score sport subscale at 6 mo ($\Delta8.4$ points), 12 mo ($\Delta9.8$ points), 30 mo ($\Delta3.7$ points)
Larson et al,[51] 2014	79	85 Hips undergoing revision arthroscopic FAI correction	• Capsular plication was significant ($P = .032$) predictor for better outcomes with revision surgery

SUMMARY

The hip capsule is a highly complex anatomic structure, which influences normal hip motion and biomechanics. The deep constrained ball-and-socket joint is completely surrounded by the inert noncontractile iliofemoral, pubofemoral, and ischiofemoral ligaments. A dynamic stabilizing capsular contribution exists in the iliocapsularis and gluteus minimus, among other musculotendinous structures crossing the joint. Variable types (interportal and T) and sizes of capsulotomy are necessary to sufficiently visualize and address bony and soft tissue pathologic source of symptoms. Unrepaired capsulotomies may leave the hip significantly unstable to variable degrees (microinstability with femoral head translation, in addition to rotation, and macroinstability, with femoral head subluxation or dislocation). Capsular closure is a necessary part of a comprehensive arthroscopic hip preservation procedure. Greater titration of the degree of plication may be performed for patients with risk factors for postoperative instability. Clinical outcomes examining the influence of capsular management in arthroscopic hip surgery is limited but demonstrates statistically significant and clinically relevant improvements at short- and midterm follow-up.

REFERENCES

1. Draovitch P, Edelstein J, Kelly BT. The layer concept: utilization in determining the pain generators, pathology and how structure determines treatment. Curr Rev Musculoskelet Med 2012;5(1):1–8.
2. Tonnis D, Heinecke A. Acetabular and femoral anteversion: relationship with osteoarthritis of the hip. J Bone Joint Surg Am 1999;81(12):1747–70.
3. Harris J, Slikker W 3rd, Gupta AK, et al. Routine complete capsular closure during hip arthroscopy. Arthrosc Tech 2013;2(2):e89–94.
4. Jackson TJ, Peterson AB, Akeda M, et al. Biomechanical effects of capsular shift in the treatment of hip microinstability: creation and testing of a novel hip instability model. Am J Sports Med 2016;44(3):689–95.
5. Abrams GD, Hart MA, Takami K, et al. Biomechanical evaluation of capsulotomy, capsulectomy, and capsular repair on hip rotation. Arthroscopy 2015;31(8):1511–7.
6. Bayne CO, Stanley R, Simon P, et al. Effect of capsulotomy on hip stability-a consideration during hip arthroscopy. Am J Orthop (Belle Mead NJ) 2014;43(4):160–5.
7. Martin HD, Savage A, Braly BA, et al. The function of the hip capsular ligaments: a quantitative report. Arthroscopy 2008;24(2):188–95.
8. Myers CA, Register BC, Lertwanich P, et al. Role of the acetabular labrum and the iliofemoral ligament in hip stability: an in vitro biplane fluoroscopy study. Am J Sports Med 2011;39(Suppl):85S–91S.
9. Hewitt JD, Glisson RR, Guilak F, et al. The mechanical properties of the human hip capsule ligaments. J Arthroplasty 2002;17(1):82–9.
10. Walters BL, Cooper JH, Rodriguez JA. New findings in hip capsular anatomy: dimensions of capsular thickness and pericapsular contributions. Arthroscopy 2014;30(10):1235–45.
11. McCormick F, Slikker W 3rd, Harris JD, et al. Evidence of capsular defect following hip arthroscopy. Knee Surg Sports Traumatol Arthrosc 2014;22(4):902–5.
12. Harris JD, Gerrie BJ, Lintner DM, et al. Microinstability of the hip and the splits radiograph. Orthopedics 2016;39(1):e169–75.

13. Mitchell RJ, Gerrie BJ, McCulloch PC, et al. Radiographic evidence of hip micro-instability in elite ballet. Arthroscopy 2016;32:1–8.

14. Duplantier NL, McCulloch PC, Nho SJ, et al. Hip dislocation or subluxation following hip arthroscopy: a systematic review. Arthroscopy 2016. [Epub ahead of print].

15. Wassilew GI, Janz V, Heller MO, et al. Real time visualization of femoroacetabular impingement and subluxation using 320-slice computed tomography. J Orthop Res 2013;31(2):275–81.

16. Harris JD, Gerrie BJ, Varner KE, et al. Radiographic prevalence of dysplasia, cam, and pincer deformities in elite ballet. Am J Sports Med 2016;44(1):20–7.

17. Philippon MJ, Briggs KK, Carlisle JC, et al. Joint space predicts THA after hip arthroscopy in patients 50 years and older. Clin Orthop Relat Res 2013;471(8): 2492–6.

18. Kocaoglu H, Başarır K, Akmeşe R, et al. The effect of traction force and hip abduction angle on pudendal nerve compression in hip arthroscopy: a cadaveric model. Arthroscopy 2015;31(10):1974–80.e6.

19. Telleria JJ, Safran MR, Harris AH, et al. Risk of sciatic nerve traction injury during hip arthroscopy-is it the amount or duration? An intraoperative nerve monitoring study. J Bone Joint Surg Am 2012;94(22):2025–32.

20. Birmingham P. Hip arthroscopy neurapraxia: is it only about weight of traction? J Bone Joint Surg Am 2012;94(22):e169.

21. Mei-Dan O, McConkey MO, Young DA. Hip arthroscopy distraction without the use of a perineal post: prospective study. Orthopedics 2013;36(1):e1–5.

22. Mei-Dan O, McConkey MO, Young DA. Improved limb positioning and hip access during hip arthroscopy with articulated traction device. Arthrosc Tech 2013;2(1): e51–4.

23. Harris JD, McCormick FM, Abrams GD, et al. Complications and reoperations during and after hip arthroscopy: a systematic review of 92 studies and more than 6,000 patients. Arthroscopy 2013;29(3):589–95.

24. Weber AE, Harris JD, Nho SJ. Complications in hip arthroscopy: a systematic re-view and strategies for prevention. Sports Med Arthrosc 2015;23(4):187–93.

25. Gupta A, Redmond JM, Hammarstedt JE, et al. Safety measures in hip arthros-copy and their efficacy in minimizing complications: a systematic review of the evidence. Arthroscopy 2014;30(10):1342–8.

26. Park MS, Yoon SJ, Kim YJ, et al. Hip arthroscopy for femoroacetabular impinge-ment: the changing nature and severity of associated complications over time. Arthroscopy 2014;30(8):957–63.

27. Byrd JW, Jones KS. Hip arthroscopy for labral pathology: prospective analysis with 10-year follow-up. Arthroscopy 2009;25(4):365–8.

28. Domb B, Hanypsiak B, Botser I. Labral penetration rate in a consecutive series of 300 hip arthroscopies. Am J Sports Med 2012;40(4):864–9.

29. Badylak JS, Keene JS. Do iatrogenic punctures of the labrum affect the clinical results of hip arthroscopy? Arthroscopy 2011;27(6):761–7.

30. Aoki SK, Beckmann JT, Wylie JD. Hip arthroscopy and the anterolateral portal: avoiding labral penetration and femoral articular injuries. Arthrosc Tech 2012; 1(2):e155–60.

31. Alpaugh K, Shin SR, Martin SD. Intra-articular fluid distension for initial portal placement during hip arthroscopy: the "femoral head drop" technique. Arthrosc Tech 2015;4(1):e23–7.

32. Konan S, Rhee SJ, Haddad FS. Hip arthroscopy: analysis of a single surgeon's learning experience. J Bone Joint Surg Am 2011;93(Suppl 2):52–6.

33. Hoppe DJ, de Sa D, Simunovic N, et al. The learning curve for hip arthroscopy: a systematic review. Arthroscopy 2014;30(3):389–97.

34. Lee YK, Ha YC, Hwang DS, et al. Learning curve of basic hip arthroscopy technique: CUSUM analysis. Knee Surg Sports Traumatol Arthrosc 2013;21(8):1940–4.

35. Mather III RC, Karas V, Federer AE, et al. Suspension technique provides superior visualization, capsular protection. Orthopedics Today 2015;1–2. Available at: http://www.healio.com/orthopedics/arthroscopy/news/print/orthopedics-today/%7B4df34e3a-d9e8-46c8-b19c-f4ed85518848%7D/suspension-technique-provides-superior-visualization-capsular-protection. Accessed July 1, 2015.

36. Thakral R, Ochiai D. Arthroscopic technique for treatment of combined pathology associated with femoroacetabular impingement syndrome using traction sutures and a minimal capsulotomy. Arthrosc Tech 2014;3(4):e527–32.

37. Chandrasekaran S, Vemula SP, Martin TJ, et al. Arthroscopic technique of capsular plication for the treatment of hip instability. Arthrosc Tech 2015;4(2):e163–7.

38. Wylie JD, Beckmann JT, Maak TG, et al. Dislocation after hip arthroscopy for cam-type femoroacetabular impingement leading to progressive arthritis. J Bone Joint Surg Case Connect 2015;5(3):e80.

39. Dierckman BD, Guanche CA. Anterior hip capsuloligamentous reconstruction for recurrent instability after hip arthroscopy. Am J Orthop (Belle Mead NJ) 2014;43(12):E319–23.

40. Austin DC, Horneff JG 3rd, Kelly JD. Anterior hip dislocation 5 months after hip arthroscopy. Arthroscopy 2014;30(10):1380–2.

41. Rosenbaum A, Roberts T, Flaherty M, et al. Posterior dislocation of the hip following arthroscopy - a case report and discussion. Bull Hosp Jt Dis (2013) 2014;72(2):181–4.

42. Sansone M, Ahldén M, Jónasson P, et al. Total dislocation of the hip joint after arthroscopy and ileopsoas tenotomy. Knee Surg Sports Traumatol Arthrosc 2013;21(2):420–3.

43. Mei-Dan O, McConkey MO, Brick M. Catastrophic failure of hip arthroscopy due to iatrogenic instability: can partial division of the ligamentum teres and iliofemoral ligament cause subluxation? Arthroscopy 2012;28(3):440–5.

44. Souza BG, Dani WS, Honda EK, et al. Do complications in hip arthroscopy change with experience? Arthroscopy 2010;26(8):1053–7.

45. Ranawat AS, McClincy M, Sekiya JK. Anterior dislocation of the hip after arthroscopy in a patient with capsular laxity of the hip. A case report. J Bone Joint Surg Am 2009;91(1):192–7.

46. Benali Y, Katthagen BD. Hip subluxation as a complication of arthroscopic debridement. Arthroscopy 2009;25(4):405–7.

47. Matsuda DK. Acute iatrogenic dislocation following hip impingement arthroscopic surgery. Arthroscopy 2009;25(4):400–4.

48. Wylie JD, Beckmann JT, Maak TG, et al. Arthroscopic capsular repair for symptomatic hip instability after previous hip arthroscopic surgery. Am J Sports Med 2016;44(1):39–45.

49. Frank RM, Lee S, Bush-Joseph CA, et al. Improved outcomes after hip arthroscopic surgery in patients undergoing T-capsulotomy with complete repair versus partial repair for femoroacetabular impingement: a comparative matched-pair analysis. Am J Sports Med 2014;42(11):2634–42.

50. Larson CM, Stone RM, Grossi EF, et al. Ehlers-Danlos syndrome: arthroscopic management for extreme soft-tissue hip instability. Arthroscopy 2015;31(12):2287–94.

51. Larson CM, Giveans MR, Samuelson KM, et al. Arthroscopic hip revision surgery for residual femoroacetabular impingement (FAI): surgical outcomes compared with a matched cohort after primary arthroscopic FAI correction. Am J Sports Med 2014;42(8):1785–90.

The Etiology and Arthroscopic Surgical Management of Cam Lesions

 CrossMark

Brian C. Werner, MD*, Michael A. Gaudiani, BA, Anil S. Ranawat, MD

KEYWORDS

- Cam-type impingement • Adolescent athletes • CT scan • Hip arthroscopy
- Femoral osteoplasty

KEY POINTS

- Arthroscopic treatment of femoroacetabular impingement (FAI) and other hip disorders is an area of rapidly developing interest in the United States.
- The etiology unknown, but recent evidence suggests a developmental etiology owing to increased stress placed on the immature physis owing to youth sports activities.
- Imaging is important in the characterization of a cam-type lesion, including plain radiographs, MRI, and often computed tomography scans for preoperative planning.
- The site for arthroscopic cam decompression is best verified by fluoroscopy, as is the extent of cam decompression.
- Short-term and mid-term outcomes for arthroscopic osteoplasty of cam lesions for isolated cam-type deformity and mixed cam-pincer FAI have been well-described and are favorable.

INTRODUCTION

Femoroacetabular impingement (FAI) syndrome is a clinical entity that until recently was poorly understood. It is characterized by hip pain associated with decreased hip range of motion owing to either femoral cam or acetabular pincer lesions or some combination thereof.[1] It affects people in their active years of life, and is considered by many to be a risk factor for the eventual development of osteoarthritis.[2,3] Accompanying these advances in the understanding of the pathophysiology and pathomechanics of FAI have been improvements in arthroscopic techniques for addressing them. Arthroscopic treatment of FAI and other hip disorders is an area of rapidly developing interest in the United States, with substantial increases in arthroscopic hip procedures being performed over the past decade.[4–7]

Department of Sports Medicine and Shoulder Service, Hospital for Special Surgery, 535 East 70th Street, New York, NY 10021, USA
* Corresponding author.
E-mail address: wernerb@hss.edu

Clin Sports Med 35 (2016) 391–404
http://dx.doi.org/10.1016/j.csm.2016.02.007
0278-5919/16/$ – see front matter © 2016 Elsevier Inc. All rights reserved.

Many hip conditions in the past that would now be considered FAI either went undetected or were misdiagnosed as chronic muscle strains. This is of particular importance in younger, athletic patients, because their risk for adverse consequences from FAI are much greater. In a recent study of athletes with chronic adductor-related groin pain, the prevalence of radiographic signs of FAI was 94%. Although the prevalence of FAI in athletes is not known, there is evidence suggesting it may be common. In football players at the National Football League Combine with a history of hip injury or hip pain, radiographic signs of FAI were present in 94.3% of hips.[8] Combined cam and pincer-type FAI was the most common (61.8%) finding compared with isolated cam (9.8%) and pincer (22.8%) FAI.[8] Morphologic abnormalities associated with FAI were also identified in the majority of hips (95%) in asymptomatic collegiate football players and about one-half of female collegiate athletes.[9,10] These numbers are actually higher than those previously reported in the general population.[11]

This article focuses on the cam lesion, including the etiology, risk factors, pathomechanics, diagnosis, surgical management, and reported outcomes after arthroscopic management.

ETIOLOGY

Cam-type deformity of the proximal femur is a relative increase, either focally or globally, in the diameter of the femoral neck compared with the femoral head.[12] This results in a structural deformity, which includes loss of the femoral head–neck offset and/or sphericity. Cam deformity can occur as an isolated finding, or more commonly, can be found in association with acetabular overcoverage (pincer lesion).

The exact etiology of the cam lesion is unknown and although the majority are considered to be idiopathic, several related conditions have been implicated in the development of abnormal proximal femoral anatomy, including slipped capital femoral epiphysis, Legg–Calve–Perthes disease, and congenital or acquired coxa vara.[12–15]

More alarming is recent evidence that suggests that certain high-impact sports participation during growth may play an important role. Three recent studies reported a significantly increased prevalence of cam-type lesions in asymptomatic adolescents participating in soccer and basketball compared with nonathlete controls.[16–18] A recent prospective study found that cam deformities gradually develop during skeletal maturation in youth soccer players and are probably stable from the time of physeal closure.[19] Numerous other studies have reported high rates of cam deformities in both asymptomatic and symptomatic athletic adults.[11,20,21] These authors all postulate that repetitive mechanical forces inherent to these athletic activities enhance the development of an osseous overgrowth.

Numerous studies have attempted to identify risk factors for the development of cam deformity. A high level of activity, including sports participation during adolescence, has been theorized to affect the immature physis and has been consistently associated with the development of cam-type deformity.[21] Nepple and colleagues[21] published a metaanalysis of 300 hips in 208 athletes compared with 290 hips in 194 nonathletes and found that high-level male athletes are 1.9 to 8.0 times more likely to develop a cam deformity than male control subjects. Siebenrock and colleagues[17] reported similar findings in a study comparing male basketball players with age-matched volunteers. The average maximum alpha angle was significantly greater in athletes (61°) compared with nonathletic controls (47°). Agricola and colleagues[19] prospectively followed 63 preprofessional soccer players and obtained radiographs to monitor for the prevalence and development of cam deformity. The authors found that, in youth soccer players, cam deformities gradually develop during skeletal maturation and are probably stable from the time of physeal closure, which led them to theorize that the formation of such deformities could be prevented by adjusting athletic activities during a small period of skeletal growth.

Sex has also been consistently implicated in the development of cam-type deformity, with males being affected nearly four times as frequently as females.[22–25] Gosvig and colleagues[23] reported that cam-type deformity was present in 19.6% of male participants and 5.2% of female participants in a study evaluating more than 3500 patients enrolled in the Copenhagen Osteoarthritis Substudy. Several recent studies have confirmed these findings and have demonstrated that females typically have radiographic findings of pincer-type FAI, including higher incidences of coxa profunda and crossover sign, whereas male patients have the described features of cam-type impingement more frequently.[12,24]

As mentioned, hip conditions in childhood and adolescence that alter the proximal femoral anatomy can also be considered risk factors for cam-type impingement, including slipped capital femoral epiphysis, Legg–Calve–Perthes disease, congenital or acquired coxa vara, and osteonecrosis.[12–15] Additional risk factors identified in other studies include race and genetics.[12]

DIAGNOSIS AND IMAGING

Obtaining a comprehensive musculoskeletal history and understanding of the patient's symptom is an important initial step in diagnosing and managing patients with potential cam deformity. Patient history and clinical evaluation and are of significant importance, because many patients have cam lesions that are not necessarily symptomatic or in need of treatment.[26]

Imaging plays essential roles in the initial diagnostic workup, further characterization of pathology, preoperative planning, and intraoperative decision making. The initial diagnostic workup for FAI, including assessment of a potential cam-type lesion, begins with standard radiographic views of the hip, including standing anteroposterior pelvis radiograph and a lateral view of the hip[27] (**Fig. 1**). The authors typically obtain a Dunn lateral view, because the diagnosis of a pathologic femoral head/neck contour depends on the radiologic projection. The Dunn view in 45° or 90° flexion or a cross-table projection in internal rotation best show femoral head/neck asphericity, whereas anteroposterior or externally rotated cross-table views are likely to miss asphericity

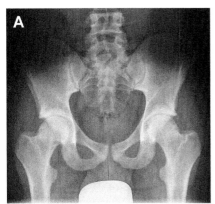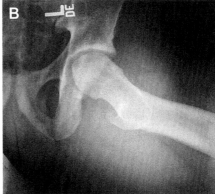

Fig. 1. Anteroposterior pelvis (*A*) and Dunn lateral (*B*) views of the left hip demonstrates findings of severe cam-type femoroacetabular impingement.

and underestimate the degree of cam deformity[28] (see **Fig. 1**B). Numerous measurements can be made on these radiographs, which are well-described and not the subject of this surgery-focused review. Depending on the clinical history and findings on physical examination and plain radiographs, MRI is often indicated, because it allows evaluation of the articular cartilage and labrum, further characterization of morphologic abnormalities of the proximal femur, and evaluation for other sources of the patients' symptoms[27] (**Fig. 2**).

Once the decision for surgical treatment is made, additional imaging can be vital for appropriate preoperative planning and intraoperative assessment and decision making. The authors routinely obtain computed tomography (CT) scans with 3-dimensional reconstructions to completely characterize the bony anatomy of the proximal femur and to plan for cam resection (**Fig. 3**). The use and importance of CT scans to evaluate cam lesions is supported by numerous recent studies.[29] Although plain radiographs have been found to correlate well with CT for the imaging of cam-type impingement, CT has been demonstrated in more recent studies to generate greater alpha angles and more accurately describe the location and topography of the lesion preoperatively.[30–32] In addition to improved accuracy in characterizing proximal femoral morphology, CT also allows better assessment of femoral version, neck–shaft angles and characterization of cam morphology. Heyworth and coauthors reported a high correlation between 3-dimensional CT findings and arthroscopic findings when used for cam-type lesions.[33]

Intraoperative imaging is also important to localize portals, plan cam resection, and confirm that adequate resection has been accomplished. Intraoperative fluoroscopy has been demonstrated as quite accurate in the assessment of cam lesions. Larson and Wulf[34] described the use of intraoperative fluoroscopy for the confirmation of cam resection. Ross and colleagues[35] compared 6 specific intraoperative fluoroscopic views with preoperative 3-dimensional CT and found that fluoroscopic imaging can be used to localize and visualize cam lesions intraoperative and conform complete

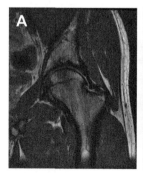 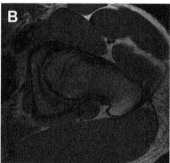 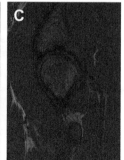

Fig. 2. Coronal (*A*), axial (*B*), and sagittal (*C*) fast-spin echo MRI of the same patient as in **Fig. 1**, demonstrating findings of severe femoroacetabular impingement with proliferative bone formation both anterior and posterior to the femoral head neck junction with insufficient offset. The femoral head has remodeled with an elliptical contour owing to severe impingement and there is diffuse abnormality in all visualized cartilage. Subchondral sclerosis and slight depression of the subchondral bone is notable where there is impending delamination of the cartilage. There is also a marginal osteophyte formation. Oblique axial images demonstrate severe coxa profunda with overcontainment of the remodeled elliptical femoral head. The anterior labrum is chronically torn. Version analysis, corrected for degree of distal femoral rotation, was also completed and demonstrated left femoral anteversion of 9.2°.

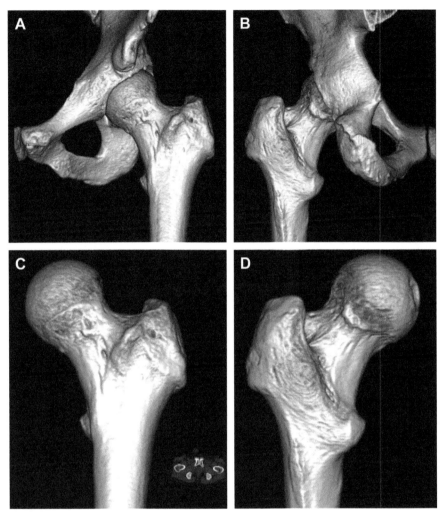

Fig. 3. Preoperative computed tomography (CT) scans of the left hip of a 35-year-old patient including the acetabulum (*A, B*) and with the pelvis subtracted (*C, D*) demonstrating loss of anterior femoral head neck offset with productive bone formation at the head neck junction. Focal productive bone formation at posterior head neck junction. Center edge angle, tonnis angle, neck shaft angle, acetabular version at 1:00, 2:00, and 3:00, alpha angle, beta angle and femoral neck anteversion were also all calculated from the CT scans.

intraoperative resection in most patients. The accuracy and reproducibility of using intraoperative fluoroscopy has led to it largely supplanting other methods of intraoperative resection confirmation, although the use of intraoperative CT scan has also been described.[36]

INDICATIONS AND CONTRAINDICATIONS

- Although little evidence exists validating nonoperative treatment of FAI, most patients with FAI are typically managed conservatively initially, including activity modification, oral antiinflammatory medications, and physical therapy, and when these fail, diagnostic and/or therapeutic intraarticular injections. These measures are not the focus of this review.

- Both open and arthroscopic approaches for resecting cam lesions have been described, although recently arthroscopic intervention has become increasingly popular. Several studies have shown no statistical difference in the amount of bony resection between open and arthroscopic methods.[37,38]
- We describe arthroscopic techniques for the treatment of cam-type deformity. The goal of this approach is to restore normal proximal femoral bony anatomy by ensuring sufficient resection of the abnormal bone that impinges on the acetabulum while avoiding neurovascular injury, inadequate resection, overresection or iatrogenic labral or chondral injury.[39]

AUTHOR'S PREFERRED SURGICAL TECHNIQUE
Preoperative Planning

- A patient indicated for surgery will typically already have appropriate plain radiographs (see **Fig. 1**) and typically also an MRI (see **Fig. 2**). When cam impingement is suspected based on examination and preoperative radiographs, the authors typically obtain a CT scan with 3-dimensional reconstructions (see **Fig. 3**) to evaluate more thoroughly the bony architecture of the proximal femoral neck, completely assess the cam lesion, and for preoperative planning.

Preparation and Patient Positioning

- The patient is laid supine on the traction table and all bony prominences are well-padded. Intravenous antibiotics are given within 1 hour of surgery and a time-out is performed before beginning the procedure.
- Using a hip distractor (Hip Positioning System, Smith & Nephew, Andover, MA), sufficient traction is placed on the ipsilateral extremity such that approximately 10 mm of distraction is present within the joint. This is verified with fluoroscopy (**Fig. 4**).

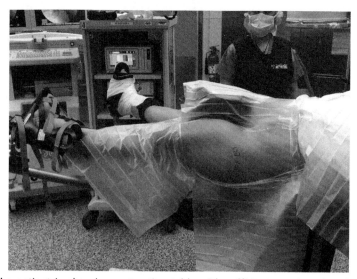

Fig. 4. The patient is placed on a traction table with sufficient traction placed such that approximately 10 mm of distraction is present within the joint.

Surgical Approach

- Portal placement can be by surgeon's preference, but the authors typically use an anterolateral portal first. A stab incision is made just superior and anterior to the greater trochanter. A curved clamp is used to bluntly dissect down to the hip capsule.
- Next a spinal needle is used to identify the correct starting point for the portal. This is done under fluoroscopic imaging. Once appropriate placement of the needle into the joint is confirmed, dilute eipinephrine solution is injection to expand the capsule, and a wire is then placed through the cannulated needle, which is then removed. A cannula is inserted over the wire and into the joint. The 70° arthroscope is then inserted through the cannula and the anterior triangle is identified.
- Under direct arthroscopic visualization, a modified mid anterior portal is made entering through the anterior triangle. The arthroscope is then inserted into the modified mid anterior portal and an arthroscopic knife is then placed through the anterolateral portal to begin the capsulotomy connecting the 2 portals. Although it varies slightly depending on patient size, the average anterolateral and mid anterior portals enter the hip at 12 o'clock and 2 o'clock, respectively, which results in an average of 3 cm between portals.

Surgical Procedure

- Diagnostic arthroscopy is completed and the pathology is confirmed.
- Typically, osteochondroplasty of a cam lesion is performed in conjunction with other procedures, which are described in other articles in this issue.
- The authors typically address any pincer, labral or chondral pathology before addressing the cam lesion, because the latter is performed without traction.
- To address the cam deformity, traction is released and the hip is flexed to approximately 20° with neutral rotation, to slight external rotation.
- Fluoroscopy is used to obtain an appropriate modified lateral radiograph that identifies the cam lesion, adjusted to best view the apex of the cam deformity (**Fig. 5**).
- The authors typically perform a "T-capsulotomy" to work in the peripheral compartment. We perform the capsulotomy by elevating the gluteus minimus

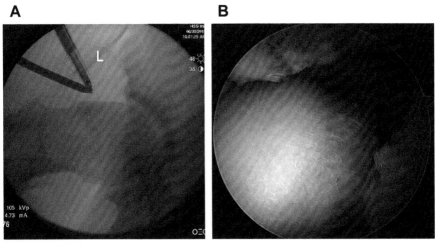

Fig. 5. (*A, B*) Fluoroscopy is used intraoperatively to identify the cam lesion, similar to the lateral view obtained preoperatively.

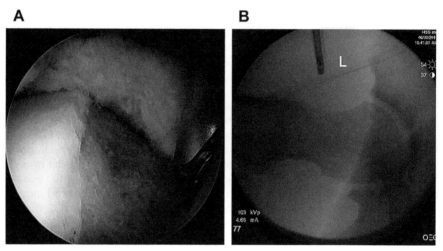

Fig. 6. Cam decompression is carried out with the use of an arthroscopic burr (*A*). Fluoroscopy is used to confirm that the decompression is complete (*B*).

and iliocapsularis off the ligament of Bigelow then incising the ligament between the medial and lateral limbs of the ligament of Bigelow.

- The retinacular vessels are identified and mark the limit of the cam decompression posterosuperiorly. These must be preserved throughout the duration of the case.
- Cam decompression is carried out with the use of an arthroscopic burr. The resection is usually from 1 o'clock to 5 o'clock, proximal up to the physeal scar and tapered distally to the neck (**Fig. 6**A). Fluoroscopy in multiple planes is used to confirm that the decompression is complete (**Fig. 6**B).
- Finally, the T portion of the capsule is closed sequentially by using a BirdBeak suture penetrator (Arthrex, Naples FLA) through the distal accessory portal and the Acupass suture passing device (Smith & Nephew) to place and tie the sutures arthroscopically. On rare occasions, the introportal cut is also repaired.
- A sterile dressing is applied as well as a hip abduction brace for most patients. A continuous passive motion machine is also started

AUTHOR'S POSTOPERATIVE CARE

- The authors place the majority of patients in a hip abduction brace for the first 2 weeks postoperatively. Range of motion is allowed in the brace from 0 to

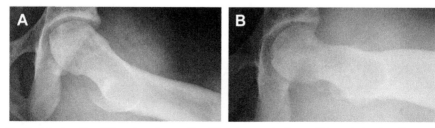

Fig. 7. Preoperative (*A*) and postoperative (*B*) anteroposterior and Dunn lateral radiographs of the 19-year-old patient from **Figs. 1** and **2** demonstrating interval cam resection of the left femur.

Table 1
Arthroscopic treatment of cam deformity: outcomes

Study	No. of Patients	Mean Age (y)	Mean Follow-up (y)	Population	Outcomes	Complications
General population						
Byrd & Jones,[43] 2009 Level IV	200	33	1.7	General population 79% isolated cam-type FAI, 21% mixed	83% of patients improved Average 20-point improvement in mHHS	1.7% complications 0.5% convert to THA 2 neuropraxia, 1 HO
Byrd & Jones,[44] 2011 Level IV	100	34	2	General population 63% isolated cam-type FAI, 19% combined	79 good to excellent results Median 21.5-point improvement in mHHS	3% complications: 2 neuropraxia, 1 HO
Palmer et al,[48] 2012 Level IV	185	40	3.8	General population 76% isolated cam-type FAI, 24% mixed	Mean improvement in NAHS of 24.1 points Significant improvement in satisfaction Improvement in VAS pain score from 6.8 to 2.7	None reported
Philipon et al,[49] 2009 Level IV	112	40.6	2.3	General population 21% isolated cam-type, 70% mixed	Mean improvement in mHHS of 24 points Median patient satisfaction was 9/10 Mean improvement in NAHS of 14 patients	10 patients underwent THA at a mean of 16 mo postoperatively
Bardakos et al,[41] 2008 Level IV	24	33	1	General population; 24 patients with cam-type deformity correction	Mean improvement in mHHS of 24 points 83% G/E results	None reported
Nepple et al,[46] 2009 Level III	25	33	Minimum of 1	General population Compared 25 patients with cam correction with 23 patients without	96% with ≥10-point mHHS improvement Mean improvement in mHHS of 25 points G/E outcomes in 92% of patients	None in cam group

(continued on next page)

Table 1
(continued)

Study	No. of Patients	Mean Age (y)	Mean Follow-up (y)	Population	Outcomes	Complications
Ilizaliturri et al,[45] 2008 Level IV	19	34	2	General population All with cam-type deformity correction	Average 7-point improvement in WOMAC	None reported
Tran et al,[50] 2013	34	16	1.2	Adolescent population All with cam-type FAI	Average 17-point improvement in mHHS Average 17-point improvement in NAHS	None reported
Brunner, et al,[42] 2009 Level IV	53	42	2.4	General, but athletic population 58% isolated cam, 42% mixed	Mean improvement in NAHS of 31 points VAS improved from 5.7 to 1.5 SFS improved from 0.78 to 1.84	None reported
Athletic population						
Nho et al,[47] 2011 Level IV	47	23	2.3	Mixed athletic 13% isolated cam-type, 30% isolated pincer, 57% mixed	Mean 20-point improvement in mHHS score Mean 13-point improvement in HOS Significant improvement in hip flexion 79% of patients returned to play	None reported
Amenabar & O'Donnell,[40] 2013 Level IV	26	22	4.1	Australian Professional Football League players 76% with cam-type FAI	96% return to professional sport Mean 14-point improvement in mHHS Mean 12-point improvement in NAHS	None reported

Abbreviations: FAI, femoroacetabular impingement; G/E, good or excellent; HO, heterotopic ossification; HOS, Hip Outcome Score; mHHS, Modified Harris Hip Score; NAHS, nonarthritic hip score; SFS, sports frequency score; THA, total arthroplasty; VAS, visual analog score; WOMAC, Western Ontario and McMaster Universities Osteoarthritis Index.

90°. Radiographs are obtained to confirm the degree of cam resection and for a baseline in the event studies are required in the future (**Fig. 7**).
- Patients without contraindications are placed on indomethacin for 4 days (for heterotopic ossification prophylaxis) followed by 4 weeks of naprosyn.
- Patients are restricted to 50% partial foot-flat weight bearing with crutches for ambulatory assistance for 2 to 3 weeks, then allowed progressively increased weight bearing.
- At 6 weeks postoperatively, patients are allowed to begin to wean crutches, progress range of motion and begin proprioception.
- At 3 months postoperatively, patients may begin light plyometrics and increase the volume and intensity of aerobic activity.
- Between 4 to 6 months, patients may return to sporting activities.

OUTCOMES

Short-term and mid-term outcomes for arthroscopic osteoplasty of cam lesions for both isolated cam-type deformity and mixed cam-pincer FAI have been well-described and are quite favorable. **Table 1** summarizes studies that report clinical outcomes after osteoplasty for cam-type deformity.[40–50]

SUMMARY

- Arthroscopic treatment of FAI and other hip disorders is an area of rapidly developing interest in the United States
- The exact etiology of the cam lesion is unknown and although the majority are considered to be idiopathic, several childhood conditions have been implicated in the development of abnormal proximal femoral anatomy
- Imaging is important in the characterization of a cam-type lesion, including plain radiographs, MRI, and often CT scans for preoperative planning.
- The site for arthroscopic cam decompression is best verified by fluoroscopy, as is the extent of cam decompression
- Short-term and mid-term outcomes for arthroscopic osteoplasty of cam lesions for both isolated cam-type deformity and mixed cam-pincer FAI have been well-described and are quite favorable.

REFERENCES

1. Ganz R, Parvizi J, Beck M, et al. Femoroacetabular impingement: a cause for osteoarthritis of the hip. Clin Orthop Relat Res 2003;417:112–20.
2. Agricola R, Waarsing JH, Arden NK, et al. Cam impingement of the hip: a risk factor for hip osteoarthritis. Nat Rev Rheumatol 2013;9:630–4.
3. Nelson AE, Stiller JL, Shi XA, et al. Measures of hip morphology are related to development of worsening radiographic hip osteoarthritis over 6 to 13 year follow-up: the Johnston County Osteoarthritis Project. Osteoarthritis Cartilage 2016;24(3):443–50.
4. Bozic KJ, Chan V, Valone FH 3rd, et al. Trends in hip arthroscopy utilization in the united states. J Arthroplasty 2013;28:140–3.
5. Colvin AC, Harrast J, Harner C. Trends in hip arthroscopy. J Bone Joint Surg Am 2012;94:e23.
6. Montgomery SR, Ngo SS, Hobson T, et al. Trends and demographics in hip arthroscopy in the united states. Arthroscopy 2013;29:661–5.

7. Sing DC, Feeley BT, Tay B, et al. Age-related trends in hip arthroscopy: a large cross-sectional analysis. Arthroscopy 2015;31(12):2307–13.e2.

8. Nepple JJ, Brophy RH, Matava MJ, et al. Radiographic findings of femoroacetabular impingement in national football league combine athletes undergoing radiographs for previous hip or groin pain. Arthroscopy 2012;28:1396–403.

9. Kapron AL, Peters CL, Aoki SK, et al. The prevalence of radiographic findings of structural hip deformities in female collegiate athletes. Am J Sports Med 2015;43:1324–30.

10. Kapron AL, Anderson AE, Peters CL, et al. Hip internal rotation is correlated to radiographic findings of cam femoroacetabular impingement in collegiate football players. Arthroscopy 2012;28:1661–70.

11. Kapron AL, Anderson AE, Aoki SK, et al. Radiographic prevalence of femoroacetabular impingement in collegiate football players: AAOS exhibit selection. J Bone Joint Surg Am 2011;93. e111(1–10).

12. Siebenrock KA, Schwab JM. The cam-type deformity–what is it: SCFE, osteophyte, or a new disease? J Pediatr Orthop 2013;33(Suppl 1):S121–5.

13. Leunig M, Casillas MM, Hamlet M, et al. Slipped capital femoral epiphysis: early mechanical damage to the acetabular cartilage by a prominent femoral metaphysis. Acta Orthop Scand 2000;71:370–5.

14. Mirkopulos N, Weiner DS, Askew M. The evolving slope of the proximal femoral growth plate relationship to slipped capital femoral epiphysis. J Pediatr Orthop 1988;8:268–73.

15. Tannast M, Hanke M, Ecker TM, et al. LCPD: reduced range of motion resulting from extra- and intraarticular impingement. Clin Orthop Relat Res 2012;470:2431–40.

16. Siebenrock KA, Kaschka I, Frauchiger L, et al. Prevalence of cam-type deformity and hip pain in elite ice hockey players before and after the end of growth. Am J Sports Med 2013;41:2308–13.

17. Siebenrock KA, Ferner F, Noble PC, et al. The cam-type deformity of the proximal femur arises in childhood in response to vigorous sporting activity. Clin Orthop Relat Res 2011;469:3229–40.

18. Agricola R, Bessems JH, Ginai AZ, et al. The development of cam-type deformity in adolescent and young male soccer players. Am J Sports Med 2012;40:1099–106.

19. Agricola R, Heijboer MP, Ginai AZ, et al. A cam deformity is gradually acquired during skeletal maturation in adolescent and young male soccer players: a prospective study with minimum 2-year follow-up. Am J Sports Med 2014;42:798–806.

20. Gerhardt MB, Romero AA, Silvers HJ, et al. The prevalence of radiographic hip abnormalities in elite soccer players. Am J Sports Med 2012;40:584–8.

21. Nepple JJ, Vigdorchik JM, Clohisy JC. What is the association between sports participation and the development of proximal femoral cam deformity? A systematic review and meta-analysis. Am J Sports Med 2015;43(11):2833–40.

22. Allen D, Beaule PE, Ramadan O, et al. Prevalence of associated deformities and hip pain in patients with cam-type femoroacetabular impingement. J Bone Joint Surg Br 2009;91:589–94.

23. Gosvig KK, Jacobsen S, Sonne-Holm S, et al. Prevalence of malformations of the hip joint and their relationship to sex, groin pain, and risk of osteoarthritis: a population-based survey. J Bone Joint Surg Am 2010;92:1162–9.

24. Yanke AB, Khair MM, Stanley R, et al. Sex differences in patients with CAM deformities with femoroacetabular impingement: 3-dimensional computed tomographic quantification. Arthroscopy 2015;31(12):2301–6.

25. Reichenbach S, Juni P, Werlen S, et al. Prevalence of cam-type deformity on hip magnetic resonance imaging in young males: a cross-sectional study. Arthritis Care Res (Hoboken) 2010;62:1319–27.

26. Ng KC, Lamontagne M, Adamczyk AP, et al. Patient-specific anatomical and functional parameters provide new insights into the pathomechanism of cam FAI. Clin Orthop Relat Res 2015;473:1289–96.

27. Fadul DA, Carrino JA. Imaging of femoroacetabular impingement. J Bone Joint Surg Am 2009;91(Suppl 1):138–43.

28. Meyer DC, Beck M, Ellis T, et al. Comparison of six radiographic projections to assess femoral head/neck asphericity. Clin Orthop Relat Res 2006;445:181–5.

29. Audenaert EA, Mahieu P, Pattyn C. Three-dimensional assessment of cam engagement in femoroacetabular impingement. Arthroscopy 2011;27:167–71.

30. Nepple JJ, Martel JM, Kim YJ, et al, ANCHOR Study Group. Do plain radiographs correlate with CT for imaging of cam-type femoroacetabular impingement? Clin Orthop Relat Res 2012;470:3313–20.

31. Milone MT, Bedi A, Poultsides L, et al. Novel CT-based three-dimensional software improves the characterization of cam morphology. Clin Orthop Relat Res 2013;471:2484–91.

32. Kang RW, Yanke AB, Espinoza Orias AA. Emerging ideas: novel 3-D quantification and classification of cam lesions in patients with femoroacetabular impingement. Clin Orthop Relat Res 2013;471:358–62.

33. Heyworth BE, Dolan MM, Nguyen JT, et al. Preoperative three-dimensional CT predicts intraoperative findings in hip arthroscopy. Clin Orthop Relat Res 2012; 470:1950–7.

34. Larson CM, Wulf CA. Intraoperative fluoroscopy for evaluation of bony resection during arthroscopic management of femoroacetabular impingement in the supine position. Arthroscopy 2009;25:1183–92.

35. Ross JR, Bedi A, Stone RM, et al. Intraoperative fluoroscopic imaging to treat cam deformities: correlation with 3-dimensional computed tomography. Am J Sports Med 2014;42:1370–6.

36. Mofidi A, Shields JS, Tan JS, et al. Use of intraoperative computed tomography scanning in determining the magnitude of arthroscopic osteochondroplasty. Arthroscopy 2011;27:1005–13.

37. Mardones R, Lara J, Donndorff A, et al. Surgical correction of "cam-type" femoroacetabular impingement: a cadaveric comparison of open versus arthroscopic debridement. Arthroscopy 2009;25:175–82.

38. Buchler L, Neumann M, Schwab JM, et al. Arthroscopic versus open cam resection in the treatment of femoroacetabular impingement. Arthroscopy 2013;29: 653–60.

39. Kweon C, Welton KL, Kelly BT, et al. Arthroscopic treatment of cam-type impingement of the hip. JBJS Reviews 2015;3(9):e3.

40. Amenabar T, O'Donnell J. Return to sport in Australian Football League footballers after hip arthroscopy and midterm outcome. Arthroscopy 2013;29: 1188–94.

41. Bardakos NV, Vasconcelos JC, Villar RN. Early outcome of hip arthroscopy for femoroacetabular impingement: the role of femoral osteoplasty in symptomatic improvement. J Bone Joint Surg Br 2008;90:1570–5.

42. Brunner A, Horisberger M, Herzog RF. Sports and recreation activity of patients with femoroacetabular impingement before and after arthroscopic osteoplasty. Am J Sports Med 2009;37:917–22.
43. Byrd JW, Jones KS. Arthroscopic femoroplasty in the management of cam-type femoroacetabular impingement. Clin Orthop Relat Res 2009;467:739–46.
44. Byrd JW, Jones KS. Arthroscopic management of femoroacetabular impingement: minimum 2-year follow-up. Arthroscopy 2011;27:1379–88.
45. Ilizaliturri VM Jr, Orozco-Rodriguez L, Acosta-Rodriguez E, et al. Arthroscopic treatment of cam-type femoroacetabular impingement: preliminary report at 2 years minimum follow-up. J Arthroplasty 2008;23:226–34.
46. Nepple JJ, Zebala LP, Clohisy JC. Labral disease associated with femoroacetabular impingement: do we need to correct the structural deformity? J Arthroplasty 2009;24:114–9.
47. Nho SJ, Magennis EM, Singh CK, et al. Outcomes after the arthroscopic treatment of femoroacetabular impingement in a mixed group of high-level athletes. Am J Sports Med 2011;39(Suppl):14S–9S.
48. Palmer DH, Ganesh V, Comfort T, et al. Midterm outcomes in patients with cam femoroacetabular impingement treated arthroscopically. Arthroscopy 2012;28: 1671–81.
49. Philipon MJ, Briggs KK, Yen YM, et al. Outcomes following hip arthroscopy for femoroacetabular impingement with associated chondrolabral dysfunction: minimum two-year follow-up. J Bone Joint Surg Br 2009;91:16–23.
50. Tran P, Pritchard M, O'Donnell J. Outcome of arthroscopic treatment for cam type femoroacetabular impingement in adolescents. ANZ J Surg 2013;83:382–6.

Pincer Impingement

Michael M. Hadeed, MD, Jourdan M. Cancienne, MD,
F. Winston Gwathmey, MD*

KEYWORDS

- Pincer impingement • Femoroacetabular impingement • Hip arthroscopy
- Subspine impingement • Os acetabuli

KEY POINTS

- Pincer impingement occurs when pathologic contact occurs between the overhanging acetabular rim and the femoral neck.
- Several morphologic variations may predispose to a pincer-type impingement mechanism.
- Successful surgery depends on a careful preoperative examination and analysis of the imaging.

INTRODUCTION

Abnormal acetabular morphologies have been recognized as a structural problem for decades. The term pincer impingement was defined in 2003 as "the result of linear contact between the acetabular rim and the femoral head-neck junction."[1] It is a subset of femoroacetabular impingement (FAI). In the ensuing decade, substantial research has been published on pincer impingement, but there remains significant controversy surrounding the diagnosis and treatment of this disorder and its associated conditions.

This article details the modern understanding of the morphology, diagnosis, and arthroscopic treatment of pincer-type femoral acetabular impingement. Many of the current controversies (listed in **Table 1**) are addressed through a review of all the currently available literature.

ACETABULAR ANATOMY

The ilium, ischium, and pubic bones come together at the triradiate cartilage, which, in addition to the acetabular cartilage, forms the acetabulum. Initially, this complex is made up largely of hyaline cartilage, which undergoes progressive ossification.[2–4] The overall shape of the acetabular complex is not thought to change appreciably as this ossification occurs.[3,5] Fusion occurs between 13 and 18 years of age, and,

Conflicts of Interest: There are no conflicts of interest or sources of funding to report.
Department of Orthopaedic Surgery, University of Virginia, PO Box 801016, Charlottesville, VA 22908, USA
* Corresponding author.
E-mail address: fwg7d@virginia.edu

Table 1	
Current controversies in pincer impingement	
Diagnosis	What is the evidence supporting the most widely used radiographic markers of pincer impingement?
Surgical Indications	What is the best treatment option for global acetabular retroversion? What is the current role of prophylactic surgery?
Technique	What are the best methods of intraoperative evaluation of acetabuloplasty? Labral considerations during acetabuloplasty?
Associated Conditions	What is the role of subspine impingement? What is the best treatment method for associated os acetabuli?

once complete, the bony socket is augmented by a layer of articular cartilage and the acetabular labrum.[2–5]

In addition to the architecture of the acetabulum, the orientation within the body plays a pivotal role in normal hip mechanics. The average anteversion of the acetabulum is 19° with a range of approximately 10° to 30°; however, any variation of the orientation of the pelvis within the body must be taken into consideration when determining this angle.[6–12] The reported normal values for acetabular inclination range from 30° to 50° with an average of approximately 39°.[10,13]

DEFINITION AND PATHOMECHANICS

Pincer impingement is the abnormal contact between the acetabular rim and the femur caused by acetabular overcoverage.[1] The overcoverage of the acetabular can further be defined as focal, global, or true retroversion of the acetabulum.[14] Global overcoverage is predominantly caused by coxa protrusio or coxa profunda. In distinction, focal rim lesions, or cephalad retroversion of the acetabulum, results in a repetitive impaction pattern injury of a normal femoral neck against an abnormal area of acetabular overcoverage. In all cases of pincer impingement, the repetitive abutment of the femoral head-neck junction on the abnormal acetabular rim leads to compression and intrasubstance tearing of the anterosuperior labrum. This condition can lead to calcification of the labrum and further impingement.

In contrast with cam impingement, there is typically less chondral delamination present with isolated pincer impingement. However, with continued abutment, a posteroinferior contrecoup pattern of cartilage loss of the femoral head and acetabulum occurs.[15,16] In clinical practice, isolated pincer impingement is rare, and the FAI is almost always caused by coexisting cam and pincer structural abnormalities.

DIAGNOSIS

The clinical signs and symptoms as well as the physical examination findings of pincer impingement are often sensitive, but not specific. Common presenting complaints can include stiffness, pain, or limited range of motion, and typical examination findings can include a positive impingement sign, or other provocative range-of-motion tests.[17] When the diagnosis is suspected, radiographic imaging is indicated. A systematic approach should be implemented when evaluating and ordering both plain films and advanced imaging. It is important to confirm that the radiograph is properly centered over the pelvis, and that there is no abnormal tilt.

Many radiographic measurements have been proposed to diagnose pincer impingement (**Table 2**). Many of these measures were developed to analyze acetabular

Table 2
Radiographic markers of pincer impingement

	Depth	Coverage	Orientation
AP Radiograph, Centered Over Pelvis			
Coxa profunda	+	—	—
Protrusion acetabuli	+	—	—
Lateral center edge angle	+	—	—
Extrusion index	+	+	—
Crossover sign	+	+	—
Posterior wall sign	+	+	—
Ischial spine sign	—	—	+
Acetabular index	—	+	+
Tonnis angle	—	—	+
Retroversion index	—	—	+
AP acetabular wall index	—	—	+
False Profile View			
Anterior center edge angle	—	+	—

Abbreviation: AP, anteroposterior.
Data from Refs.[19–22]

dysplasia. Numerous review articles on the radiographic evaluation of FAI have been published, but the use of these measures remains controversial. Furthermore, many of the measurements now associated with pincer impingement are observed in a significant percentage of the asymptomatic population.[18] The most widely used radiographic measures include the crossover sign, posterior wall sign, and anterior and lateral center edge angle.

The radiographic diagnosis of pincer impingement is an active area of research. New methods to evaluate disorders are being developed, such as the anterior rim angle, anterior wall angle, and anterior margin ratio.[23] These new methods show promise, but will require further research to determine their clinical applicability and reliability.

SURGICAL INDICATIONS

The nonsurgical treatment of FAI focuses on improving femoroacetabular mechanics and reducing repetitive impingement and inflammation. Conservative strategies include activity modification, antiinflammatories, core and abductor strengthening, and hip motion exercises.[24,25] The decision to pursue operative intervention is based on the patient's history, physical examination, imaging, failure of conservative therapies, and temporary relief following injection.[26]

Successful treatment of any FAI requires a comprehensive approach to the osseous deformity, labral injury, and articular damage. The goals of surgical intervention are to eliminate the cause of contact between the acetabulum and femoral head-neck, and to repair any labral or articular damage that has occurred.

There are many difficulties in addressing pincer morphology with hip arthroscopy, and the global overcoverage deformities may not be amenable to arthroscopic treatment with the current techniques and tools. The most common procedure performed is acetabular rim trimming for focal overcoverage.

Global Acetabular Retroversion

In the normal hip the acetabulum is oriented anterolaterally in the sagittal plane and progresses in a reverse spiral from caudal to cranial.[27] In the retroverted hip, the opening of the acetabulum is directed in a more posterolateral direction, and the spiral is lost.[28] Acetabular retroversion has been reported in up to 20% of patients undergoing total hip arthroplasty for osteoarthritis, 17% of patients with developmental hip dysplasia, and in 5% of the general population.[28–30] Both the crossover sign and prominence of the ischial spine sign are useful in diagnosing and measuring retroversion.[28,31] The posterior wall sign is particularly important for guiding treatment in the setting of acetabular retroversion. This sign is present when the center of rotation of the femoral head is lateral to the contour of the posterior wall, and indicates a lack of posterior coverage (**Fig. 1**).

An anteverting or reverse periacetabular osteotomy (PAO) instead of arthroscopic rim trimming may be required in some cases of acetabular retroversion to avoid iatrogenic global hip instability.[27] Removing anterior rim leads to loss of acetabular volume and hip stability may be compromised. In contrast, a reverse PAO should not be performed with excessive posterior wall coverage because this could lead to posterior impingement with extension and external rotation.

The ideal candidates for reverse PAO are nonobese patients younger than 40 years with Tonnis grade changes of 0 or 1, positive posterior wall signs, and minimal to no cartilage degeneration on MRI in the area of acetabular overcoverage.[27] Siebenrock and colleagues[32] reported on the largest series of reverse PAO for correction of acetabular retroversion. Twenty-nine PAOs were performed in 22 patients with an average follow-up of 30 months. The average Merle D'Aubigné hip score improved from 14 to 16.9 points, and 28 hips had a good or excellent result, with no patients showing osteoarthritis on postoperative radiographs.

Role of Prophylactic Surgery

Positive radiographic findings that indicate pincer impingement do not necessarily indicate symptomatic disorder. However, FAI has been linked to chondrolabral

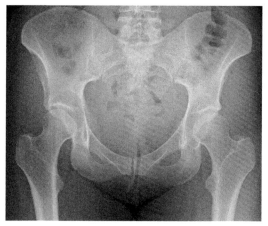

Fig. 1. Anteroposterior (AP) pelvis radiograph showing pincer-type morphology. However, note that the center of rotation of the femoral head is well lateral to the posterior wall, indicating global acetabular retroversion.

damage and the subsequent development of osteoarthritis. Recently, the question has been asked whether or not there is a role for prophylactic surgery.

Collins and colleagues[33] performed a systematic review of the literature to determine the answer to that question. The investigators ultimately stated that there was a lack of evidence to support surgical intervention in clinically asymptomatic patients. There was concern that recommending this practice could potentially expose millions of people to unnecessary surgery; up to 80% of the total number of procedures. However, they did recognize a certain situation in which the benefits may outweigh the risks. Patients who have had a prior total hip arthroplasty in the contralateral hip and radiographic evidence of FAI may benefit from a prophylactic surgery. Based on their report, it seems that up to 20% of patients may significantly benefit from prophylactic surgery.

There is theory to support prophylactic surgery; however, the currently published literature does not support this practice. In the near future, clinicians may be able to better delineate which patients may benefit from arthroscopic acetabuloplasty to the point at which prophylactic surgery is a reality. As new data emerge, it is sure to remain a topic of debate.

ARTHROSCOPIC ACETABULOPLASTY

The goal of operative intervention is to relieve the patients' symptoms by correcting the disorders causing their complaints. It is important to keep in mind the likely long-term clinical course, and what treatment will result in the best long-term outcome for the patient. When pincer impingement was first described by Ganz and colleagues,[1] the proposed treatment was surgical dislocation of the hip and open debridement of the defects. With the further development of arthroscopic tools and techniques, hip arthroscopy has seen an increase in use when addressing these deformities. However, there remain deformities that are not amenable to arthroscopic treatment.[25] When determining the appropriate management for a patient it is imperative to take an individualized approach.

Preoperative Analysis

Although the limitations of the current radiographic measures were discussed earlier, they remain the standard for evaluating the amount of acetabular rim to resect. The crossover sign and posterior wall sign are binary measures that help to determine retroversion (**Table 3**). The lateral and anterior center edge angles are more precise values that can act as a guide both preoperatively and intraoperatively. Normal values are shown in **Table 4**. Significant deviations from these normal values may indicate overcoverage that may be amenable to arthroscopic resection.

Portal Placement/Arthroscopic Orientation

When focal overcoverage is implicated in pincer impingement syndromes, it is most commonly found on the anterior portion of the acetabulum, which is treated with anterior

Table 3 Differentiating between cephalad retroversion versus true retroversion			
	Crossover Sign	Posterior Wall Sign	Prominent Ischial Sign
True retroversion	+	+	+
Cephalad retroversion	+	−	−

From Bedi A, Kelly BT. Femoroacetabular impingement. J Bone Joint Surg Am 2013;95(1):82–92.

Table 4		
Normal values for the lateral and anterior center edge angles		
Measure	**Type of Radiograph**	**Normal Values**
Lateral center edge angle	AP pelvis	34°[34]
Anterior center edge angle	False profile view	33°[35]

acetabular rim trimming. Many different portals have been described for hip arthroscopy, and ultimately the portals used are based on surgeon preference.[36] However, recent literature describes the anterolateral and anterior portals as the most appropriate and useful when attempting an anterior acetabular rim trimming procedure.[37,38]

In addition to portal choice, arthroscopic orientation is critical to a successful operation. Several methods have been described, including the clock-face method, in which the transverse acetabular ligament is at the 6 o'clock position.[38] There was concern that it was impossible to visualize the landmark for the clock face and so other orientation methods were developed. A geographic zone method was described, which was more reproducible than the clock face method, but there were concerns that it was less intuitive.[39,40] A recent cadaveric study described using the superior margin of the anterior labral sulcus as a reliable landmark to base the clock face.[40] Whichever method is used, it is imperative to have an exact measure of the acetabulum before resection.

Intraoperative Evaluation

The effects of acetabular rim trimming are difficult to visualize dynamically during arthroscopic acetabuloplasty.[41] It is essential to have a preoperative plan developed by careful review of the diagnostic imaging, and to then be able to correlate that with intraoperative fluoroscopic images and direct visualization in order to assess the progression of rim resection (**Fig. 2**). A key to adequately quantify the resection is a comfort level directing the radiology technicians in the appropriate positioning for the various radiographic views, some of which were discussed briefly earlier. It is vital to understand the nuances of hip imaging so that any image distortion does not lead to over-resection or under-resection.

The amount of acetabular rim resection in millimeters has been shown to correlate with changes in the lateral center edge angle preoperatively and postoperatively.[42] Prospective data were collected that showed that 1 mm of resection at the 12 o'clock

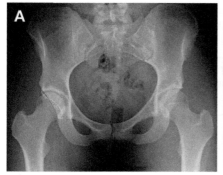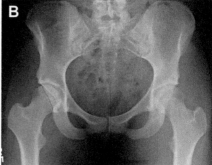

Fig. 2. (*A*) Crossover sign indicating pincer-type morphology shown on a preoperative AP radiograph. (*B*) Postoperative AP radiograph showing correction of crossover sign. (*Blue line* shows the posterior wall of the acetabulum. *Yellow line* shows the anterior wall of the acetabulum.)

position equaled 2.4° of change, and 5 mm of resection correlated with 5° of change.[42] A formula was proposed to calculate the exact change over time so that any amount of resection can be converted to a change in the radiograph and vice versa. These data allow arthroscopists to actively monitor the amount of rim resection being performed during a procedure.

Newer data suggest that it is beneficial to use the anterior center edge angle as opposed to the more traditional lateral center edge angle.[43] Most rim resection done for pincer impingement happens on the anterior aspect of the acetabulum, which is better captured with this view. Kling and colleagues[43] showed that the change over time in the anterior center edge angle is more linear per millimeter of rim resected. Furthermore, the change was magnified, which made it more precise. Change over time may have an advantage as an intraoperative monitor of resection.

MANAGEMENT OF THE ACETABULAR LABRUM

The nature of pincer impingement is abnormal bony contact; however, the labrum lies between those points of contact, and a preoperative plan to address it is necessary when undertaking this procedure. When hip arthroscopy was first established as a viable method to address pincer morphology, it was typical to simply debride/excise the labrum along with the bony overgrowth. However, as techniques evolved, more surgeons began to refix the labrum once a bony resection was completed.[16]

Refix Versus Resect

The first article to address this issue in patients undergoing purely arthroscopic treatment of pincer impingement was published in 2009 by Larson and Giveans.[44] The investigators retrospectively reviewed cases of both labral debridement and labral repair during acetabuloplasty. The labral debridement group was retrospectively evaluated, and based on intraoperative images was limited to only those patients who would have been eligible for labral repair if the techniques had been in practice at that time. Although both groups showed overall improvement, compared with each other, the labral repair group had significantly better patient-reported outcome scores as well as a greater percentage of good to excellent results. There were limitations, but this provided reasonably strong evidence that labral repair may be advantageous when possible. A subsequent article published by the Larson and colleagues[45] in 2012 expanded on the results of the previous study. This article tracked the same 2 groups of patients over a longer follow-up period of 3.5 years. The results of this study showed a durable difference between the two groupings.

In 2013 a prospective randomized study was published by Krych and colleagues[46] comparing labral repair versus debridement. As was seen in previous studies, those patients who underwent labral repair had better outcomes than those who underwent labral debridement. Based on these studies, and the absence of literature to the contrary, it seems that, whenever possible, the labrum should be salvaged and refixed after appropriate resection of the bony overgrowth.

Labral Detachment During Acetabuloplasty

Once it was determined that refixing the labrum was preferable to pure debridement, different techniques began to evolve. Classically, the labrum was detached to expose the acetabular rim.[38] However, recent investigations have begun to assess whether it is better to preserve the chondrolabral junction when possible (**Fig. 3**). Redmond and colleagues[47] compared the two techniques and found no difference in outcomes at

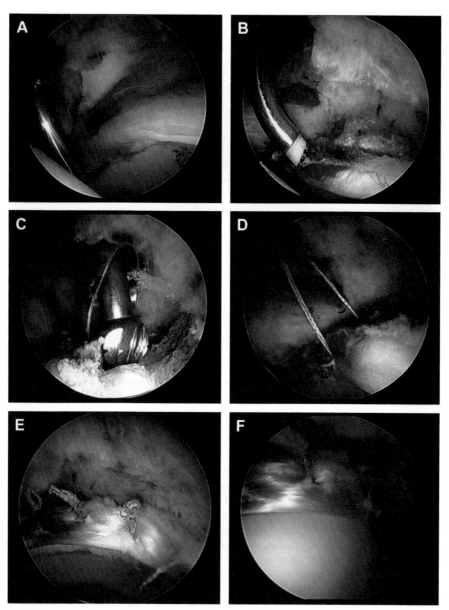

Fig. 3. Intraoperative arthroscopic views of pincer deformity correction. (*A*) Labral erythema and intrasubstance tearing indicates a pincer-type mechanism. (*B*) Labrum reflected from acetabular rim to expose the pincer lesion. (*C*) Acetabuloplasty to remove the overhanging bony rim contributing to the impingement mechanism. (*D*) Labral refixation with vertical mattress-type suture configuration. (*E*) Final picture of labral repair. (*F*) The labral seal is reestablished once traction is released.

2 years. In the report, the investigators elevated the capsule off the acetabular rim using electrocautery and then refixed the labrum with suture anchors once the rim resection was complete. At this point, the data do not suggest that one method is preferable to the other.

The labrum has proved to serve a critical role in maintaining normal hip joint mechanics. When possible it is preferable to preserve it as long as possible to adequately treat the bony disorder. No single mechanism of preservation has proved superior.

SUBSPINE IMPINGEMENT

Deformities of the anterior-inferior iliac spine (AIIS) are thought to be sequelae of avulsion fractures of the direct head of the rectus femoris.[48,49] As the fracture heals, hypertrophy of the AIIS can occur (**Fig. 4**). This condition can cause pain and decreased range of motion. In early case reports, the abnormalities were noticed on anteroposterior (AP) pelvis radiographs and confirmed on computed tomography (CT) images.[48,49] Because this is an extra-articular source of impingement, symptoms may not resolve after local anesthetic administration into the joint.[50] In addition, patients report pain with palpation of the AIIS.[48,51] A classification system of the defects has been proposed by Hetsroni and colleagues[52] and is shown in **Table 5**. Although reports have small sample sizes, this condition has been associated with cam deformities of the femur. The cam deformity was often recognized and treated, but the patients' symptoms persisted. Once the AIIS was debrided, the symptoms resolved.[50]

A systematic review of the literature recently summarized the current evidence behind treatment of extra-articular impingement syndromes.[51] The largest case series to date, of 163 hips, showed that, because of the broad origin of the rectus femoris on the AIIS, it was possible to safely debride the AIIS without causing clinical weakness in the rectus femoris postoperatively.[53] In an anatomic study, a bare area was identified of the AIIS anteriorly and inferiorly and was deemed a safe zone of resection.[53] A recent cadaveric study showed that the debridement of more than 10 mm from the AIIS could potentially compromise the rectus femoris origin, and surgeons should be aware of this limit when operating on subspine impingement.[54]

OS ACETABULI

Os acetabuli have been recognized as unfused secondary ossification centers of the acetabulum (**Fig. 5**). In dysplastic hips, it is thought that fragments appearing to be os

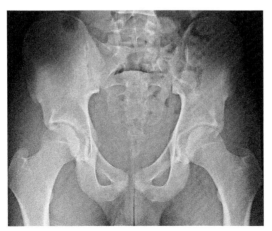

Fig. 4. AP pelvis radiograph showing a deformity of the left AIIS that may lead to subspine impingement.

Table 5
Subspine impingement classification system

Type	Description
I	Smooth ilium wall between the AIIS and the acetabular rim
II	AIIS extended to the level of the rim
III	AIIS extended distally to the acetabular rim

From Hetsroni I, Poultsides L, Bedi A, et al. Anterior inferior iliac spine morphology correlates with hip range of motion: a classification system and dynamic model. Clin Orthop Relat Res 2013;471(8):2497–503.

acetabuli are actually caused by fatigue fractures of the acetabular rim.[55] With the recognition of femoroacetabular impingement syndrome, it has been theorized that there could be a similar fatigue fracture seen in association with this condition.[55] However, at this time, it is unknown whether the fragments seen in association with femoroacetabular impingement are caused by abnormal acetabular development or by fatigue fractures from the impingement mechanism.[55,56]

The best method of treatment is unknown, but likely should be assessed on a case-by-case basis. Advanced imaging can be helpful to the surgeon when determining how to treat the fragment (either by resection or internal fixation).[57] The concern with complete resection is that the hip will then become unstable.[58,59] Several case reports have proposed a method of internal fixation in which the head of the screw is then covered by the reattached labrum.[56,60] If the fragment is amenable to this type of procedure, it seems to have good outcomes, albeit in a limited sample size.[56,60]

These associated conditions are important to be aware of when evaluating patients with possible pincer impingement. A thorough history, physical examination, and radiographic evaluation show the disorder involved in the patient's complaints only

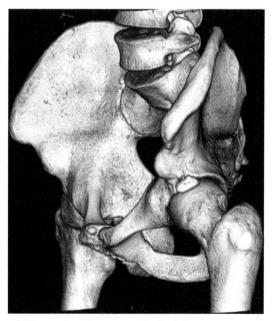

Fig. 5. Reconstructed CT scan showing os acetabuli of the anterosuperior acetabular rim.

if the surgeon is aware of all possibilities and is able to correlate the anatomy with the symptoms.

COMPLICATIONS

Although complications of hip arthroscopy are uncommon, several have been reported in the literature, including but not limited to neurapraxias, intra-abdominal fluid extravasation, cartilage scuffing, and instrument breakage.[61] Those complications specific to pincer impingement include the sequelae of both under-resection (incomplete reshaping) and over-resection (edge loading and iatrogenic hip instability) of the acetabular rim.

There is a fine line between resecting the appropriate amount of acetabulum to rectify the patient's symptoms and making sure that the remaining structure is significant enough to allow for a long-term stable articulation. Minor to moderate over-resection can lead to edge loading of the acetabulum, whereas more severe over-resection can lead to gross hip instability. The latter condition is exceedingly rare but catastrophic.[61] Because of concern for those complications, it is much more common to witness inadequate acetabuloplasty. In the absence of labral and articular damage, the leading cause of persistent pain in patients undergoing hip arthroscopy is incomplete decompression of the impinging lesion.[62,63] Adequate preoperative evaluation with radiographs as well as advanced imaging and proper intraoperative monitoring of the resection as described earlier can help prevent both of these complications.[61]

SUMMARY

Acetabular abnormalities play a large role in impingement at the hip joint. Hip arthroscopy is a growing field that has shown promise in treating pincer impingement and associated conditions. More research is needed so that clinicians can continue to refine their techniques and procedures.

REFERENCES

1. Ganz R, Parvizi J, Beck M, et al. Femoroacetabular impingement: a cause for osteoarthritis of the hip. Clin Orthop Relat Res 2003;(417):112–20.
2. Liporace FA, Ong B, Mohaideen A, et al. Development and injury of the triradiate cartilage with its effects on acetabular development: review of the literature. J Trauma 2003;54(6):1245–9.
3. Ponseti IV. Growth and development of the acetabulum in the normal child. anatomical, histological, and roentgenographic studies. J Bone Joint Surg Am 1978;60(5):575–85.
4. Weiner LS, Kelley MA, Ulin RI, et al. Development of the acetabulum and hip: computed tomography analysis of the axial plane. J Pediatr Orthop 1993;13(4): 421–5.
5. Bucholz RW, Ezaki M, Ogden JA. Injury to the acetabular triradiate physeal cartilage. J Bone Joint Surg Am 1982;64(4):600–9.
6. Anda S, Svenningsen S, Grontvedt T, et al. Pelvic inclination and spatial orientation of the acetabulum. A radiographic, computed tomographic and clinical investigation. Acta Radiol 1990;31(4):389–94.
7. McKibbin B. Anatomical factors in the stability of the hip joint in the newborn. J Bone Joint Surg Br 1970;52(1):148–59.
8. Reikeras O, Bjerkreim I, Kolbenstvedt A. Anteversion of the acetabulum and femoral neck in normals and in patients with osteoarthritis of the hip. Acta Orthop Scand 1983;54(1):18–23.

9. Siebenrock KA, Kalbermatten DF, Ganz R. Effect of pelvic tilt on acetabular retroversion: a study of pelves from cadavers. Clin Orthop Relat Res 2003;(407): 241–8.

10. Stem ES, O'Connor MI, Kransdorf MJ, et al. Computed tomography analysis of acetabular anteversion and abduction. Skeletal Radiol 2006;35(6):385–9.

11. Tonnis D, Heinecke A. Acetabular and femoral anteversion: relationship with osteoarthritis of the hip. J Bone Joint Surg Am 1999;81(12):1747–70.

12. van Bosse HJ, Lee D, Henderson ER, et al. Pelvic positioning creates error in CT acetabular measurements. Clin Orthop Relat Res 2011;469(6):1683–91.

13. Fowkes LA, Petridou E, Zagorski C, et al. Defining a reference range of acetabular inclination and center-edge angle of the hip in asymptomatic individuals. Skeletal Radiol 2011;40(11):1427–34.

14. Bedi A, Kelly BT, Khanduja V. Arthroscopic hip preservation surgery: current concepts and perspective. Bone Joint J 2013;95B(1):10–9.

15. Bedi A, Dolan M, Leunig M, et al. Static and dynamic mechanical causes of hip pain. Arthroscopy 2011;27(2):235–51.

16. Espinosa N, Beck M, Rothenfluh DA, et al. Treatment of femoro-acetabular impingement: preliminary results of labral refixation. surgical technique. J Bone Joint Surg Am 2007;89(Suppl 2 Pt 1):36–53.

17. Nepple JJ, Prather H, Trousdale RT, et al. Clinical diagnosis of femoroacetabular impingement. J Am Acad Orthop Surg 2013;21(Suppl 1):S16–9.

18. Laborie LB, Lehmann TG, Engesaeter IO, et al. Prevalence of radiographic findings thought to be associated with femoroacetabular impingement in a population-based cohort of 2081 healthy young adults. Radiology 2011;260(2):494–502.

19. Clohisy JC, Carlisle JC, Beaule PE, et al. A systematic approach to the plain radiographic evaluation of the young adult hip. J Bone Joint Surg Am 2008; 90(Suppl 4):47–66.

20. Nepple JJ, Prather H, Trousdale RT, et al. Diagnostic imaging of femoroacetabular impingement. J Am Acad Orthop Surg 2013;21(Suppl 1):S20–6.

21. Tannast M, Hanke MS, Zheng G, et al. What àre the radiographic reference values for acetabular under- and overcoverage? Clin Orthop Relat Res 2015; 473(4):1234–46.

22. Tannast M, Siebenrock KA, Anderson SE. Femoroacetabular impingement: radiographic diagnosis–what the radiologist should know. AJR Am J Roentgenol 2007; 188(6):1540–52.

23. Hellman MD, Gross CE, Hart M, et al. Radiographic comparison of anterior acetabular rim morphology between pincer femoroacetabular impingement and control. Arthroscopy 2016;32(3):468–72.

24. Bedi A, Kelly BT. Femoroacetabular impingement. J Bone Joint Surg Am 2013; 95(1):82–92.

25. Jaberi FM, Parvizi J. Hip pain in young adults: femoroacetabular impingement. J Arthroplasty 2007;22(7 Suppl 3):37–42.

26. Nepple JJ, Byrd JW, Siebenrock KA, et al. Overview of treatment options, clinical results, and controversies in the management of femoroacetabular impingement. J Am Acad Orthop Surg 2013;21(Suppl 1):S53–8.

27. Sierra RJ. The management of acetabular retroversion with reverse periacetabular osteotomy. Instr Course Lect 2013;62:305–13.

28. Reynolds D, Lucas J, Klaue K. Retroversion of the acetabulum: a cause of hip pain. J Bone Joint Surg Br 1999;81(2):281–8.

29. Li PL, Ganz R. Morphologic features of congenital acetabular dysplasia: one in six is retroverted. Clin Orthop Relat Res 2003;416:245–53.

30. Mast JW, Brunner RL, Zebrack J. Recognizing acetabular version in the radiographic presentation of hip dysplasia. Clin Orthop Relat Res 2004;418:48–53.
31. Kalberer F, Sierra RJ, Madan SS, et al. Ischial spine projection into the pelvis: a new sign for acetabular retroversion. Clin Orthop Relat Res 2008;466(3):677–83.
32. Siebenrock KA, Schoeniger R, Ganz R. Anterior femoro-acetabular impingement due to acetabular retroversion: treatment with periacetabular osteotomy. J Bone Joint Surg AM 2003;85(2):278–86.
33. Collins JA, Ward JP, Youm T. Is prophylactic surgery for femoroacetabular impingement indicated? A systematic review. Am J Sports Med 2014;42(12): 3009–15.
34. Werner CM, Ramseier LE, Ruckstuhl T, et al. Normal values of Wiberg's lateral center-edge angle and Lequesne's acetabular index–a coxometric update. Skeletal Radiol 2012;41(10):1273–8.
35. Crockarell JR Jr, Trousdale RT, Guyton JL. The anterior centre-edge angle. A cadaver study. J Bone Joint Surg Br 2000;82(4):532–4.
36. Byrd JW, Pappas JN, Pedley MJ. Hip arthroscopy: an anatomic study of portal placement and relationship to the extra-articular structures. Arthroscopy 1995; 11(4):418–23.
37. McCormick F, Federer A, Nho S. Chapter 54: Surgical technique: arthroscopic labral management. In: Nho S, Leunig M, Larson C, et al, editors. Hip arthroscopy and hip joint preservation surgery. Verlag (NY): Springer; 2015. p. 713–20. http://dx.doi.org/10.1007/978-1-4614-6965-0_57.
38. Philippon MJ, Stubbs AJ, Schenker ML, et al. Arthroscopic management of femoroacetabular impingement: osteoplasty technique and literature review. Am J Sports Med 2007;35(9):1571–80.
39. Ilizaliturri VM Jr, Byrd JW, Sampson TG, et al. A geographic zone method to describe intra-articular pathology in hip arthroscopy: cadaveric study and preliminary report. Arthroscopy 2008;24(5):534–9.
40. Philippon MJ, Michalski MP, Campbell KJ, et al. An anatomical study of the acetabulum with clinical applications to hip arthroscopy. J Bone Joint Surg Am 2014; 96(20):1673–82.
41. Zumstein M, Hahn F, Sukthankar A, et al. How accurately can the acetabular rim be trimmed in hip arthroscopy for pincer-type femoral acetabular impingement: a cadaveric investigation. Arthroscopy 2009;25(2):164–8.
42. Philippon MJ, Wolff AB, Briggs KK, et al. Acetabular rim reduction for the treatment of femoroacetabular impingement correlates with preoperative and postoperative center-edge angle. Arthroscopy 2010;26(6):757–61.
43. Kling S, Karns MR, Gebhart J, et al. The effect of acetabular rim recession on anterior acetabular coverage: a cadaveric study using the false-profile radiograph. Am J Sports Med 2015;43(4):957–64.
44. Larson CM, Giveans MR. Arthroscopic debridement versus refixation of the acetabular labrum associated with femoroacetabular impingement. Arthroscopy 2009;25(4):369–76.
45. Larson CM, Giveans MR, Stone RM. Arthroscopic debridement versus refixation of the acetabular labrum associated with femoroacetabular impingement: mean 3.5-year follow-up. Am J Sports Med 2012;40(5):1015–21.
46. Krych AJ, Thompson M, Knutson Z, et al. Arthroscopic labral repair versus selective labral debridement in female patients with femoroacetabular impingement: a prospective randomized study. Arthroscopy 2013;29(1):46–53.
47. Redmond JM, El Bitar YF, Gupta A, et al. Arthroscopic acetabuloplasty and labral refixation without labral detachment. Am J Sports Med 2015;43(1):105–12.

48. Larson CM, Kelly BT, Stone RM. Making a case for anterior inferior iliac spine/subspine hip impingement: three representative case reports and proposed concept. Arthroscopy 2011;27(12):1732–7.

49. Pan H, Kawanabe K, Akiyama H, et al. Operative treatment of hip impingement caused by hypertrophy of the anterior inferior iliac spine. J Bone Joint Surg Br 2008;90(5):677–9.

50. Sutter R, Pfirrmann CW. Atypical hip impingement. AJR Am J Roentgenol 2013; 201(3):W437–42.

51. de Sa D, Alradwan H, Cargnelli S, et al. Extra-articular hip impingement: a systematic review examining operative treatment of psoas, subspine, ischiofemoral, and greater trochanteric/pelvic impingement. Arthroscopy 2014;30(8):1026–41.

52. Hetsroni I, Poultsides L, Bedi A, et al. Anterior inferior iliac spine morphology correlates with hip range of motion: a classification system and dynamic model. Clin Orthop Relat Res 2013;471(8):2497–503.

53. Hapa O, Bedi A, Gursan O, et al. Anatomic footprint of the direct head of the rectus femoris origin: cadaveric study and clinical series of hips after arthroscopic anterior inferior iliac spine/subspine decompression. Arthroscopy 2013; 29(12):1932–40.

54. El-Shaar R, Stanton M, Biehl S, et al. Effect of subspine decompression on rectus femoris integrity and iliopsoas excursion: a cadaveric study. Arthroscopy 2015; 31(10):1903–8.

55. Martinez AE, Li SM, Ganz R, et al. Os acetabuli in femoro-acetabular impingement: stress fracture or unfused secondary ossification centre of the acetabular rim? Hip Int 2006;16(4):281–6.

56. Larson CM, Stone RM. The rarely encountered rim fracture that contributes to both femoroacetabular impingement and hip stability: a report of 2 cases of arthroscopic partial excision and internal fixation. Arthroscopy 2011;27(7): 1018–22.

57. Chhabra A, Nordeck S, Wadhwa V, et al. Femoroacetabular impingement with chronic acetabular rim fracture - 3D computed tomography, 3D magnetic resonance imaging and arthroscopic correlation. World J Orthop 2015;6(6):498–504.

58. Benali Y, Katthagen BD. Hip subluxation as a complication of arthroscopic debridement. Arthroscopy 2009;25(4):405–7.

59. Matsuda DK. Acute iatrogenic dislocation following hip impingement arthroscopic surgery. Arthroscopy 2009;25(4):400–4.

60. Rafols C, Monckeberg JE, Numair J. Unusual bilateral rim fracture in femoroacetabular impingement. Case Rep Orthop 2015;2015:210827.

61. Ilizaliturri VM Jr. Complications of arthroscopic femoroacetabular impingement treatment: a review. Clin Orthop Relat Res 2009;467(3):760–8.

62. Bogunovic L, Gottlieb M, Pashos G, et al. Why do hip arthroscopy procedures fail? Clin Orthop Relat Res 2013;471(8):2523–9.

63. Ricciardi BF, Fields K, Kelly BT, et al. Causes and risk factors for revision hip preservation surgery. Am J Sports Med 2014;42(11):2627–33.

Iliopsoas
Pathology, Diagnosis, and Treatment

Christian N. Anderson, MD

KEYWORDS

- Iliopsoas • Psoas • Coxa saltans interna • Snapping hip • Iliopsoas bursitis
- Iliopsoas tendinitis • Iliopsoas impingement

KEY POINTS

- The iliopsoas musculotendinous unit is a powerful hip flexor used for normal lower extremity function, but disorders of the iliopsoas can be a significant source of groin pain in the athletic population.
- Arthroscopic release of the iliopsoas tendon and treatment of coexisting intra-articular abnormality is effective for patients with painful iliopsoas snapping or impingement that is refractory to conservative treatment.
- Tendon release has been described at 3 locations: in the central compartment, the peripheral compartment, and at the lesser trochanter, with similar outcomes observed between the techniques.
- Releasing the tendon lengthens the musculotendinous unit, resulting in transient hip flexor weakness that typically resolves by 3 to 6 months postoperatively.

INTRODUCTION

The iliopsoas musculotendinous unit is a powerful hip flexor that is important for normal hip strength and function. Even so, pathologic conditions of the iliopsoas have been implicated as a significant source of anterior hip pain. Iliopsoas disorders have been shown to be the primary cause of chronic groin pain in 12% to 36% of athletes and are observed in 25% to 30% of athletes presenting with an acute groin injury.[1-4] Described pathologic conditions include iliopsoas bursitis, tendonitis, impingement, and snapping. Acute trauma may result in injury to the musculotendinous unit or avulsion fracture of the lesser trochanter. Developing an understanding of the anatomy and function of the musculotendinous unit is necessary to accurately determine the diagnosis and formulate an appropriate treatment strategy for disorders of the iliopsoas.

Disclosure: The author has nothing to disclose.
Tennessee Orthopaedic Alliance, The Lipscomb Clinic, Saint Thomas West Hospital, Medical Plaza East, Suite 1000, 4230 Harding Road, Nashville, TN 37205, USA
E-mail address: andersoncn@toa.com

Clin Sports Med 35 (2016) 419–433
http://dx.doi.org/10.1016/j.csm.2016.02.009
0278-5919/16/$ – see front matter © 2016 Elsevier Inc. All rights reserved.

ANATOMY AND FUNCTION

The iliopsoas tendon-muscle complex is composed of 3 muscles: the iliacus, psoas major, and psoas minor (**Fig. 1**).[5] The psoas major is a long fusiform muscle that originates on the vertebral bodies, transverse processes, and intervertebral disks of T12-L5.[5,6] The iliacus is a triangular fan-shaped muscle that is composed of medial and lateral bundles and originates from the ventral lip of the iliac crest, superior two-thirds of the iliac fossa, and sacral ala.[5–8] A third, smaller bundle, known as the ilio-infratrochanteric muscle, has been observed lateral to the lateral iliacus.[8,9] Innervation of the psoas major and iliacus are from the ventral rami of L1-3 and femoral nerve (L1-2), respectively.[5]

The psoas major and iliacus muscles converge at the level of the L5 to S2 vertebrae to form the iliopsoas muscle.[9] Before this convergence, the psoas major tendon originates above the level of the inguinal ligament from within the center of the psoas major muscle.[9] As the tendon courses distally, it rotates clockwise (right hip) and migrates posteriorly within the muscle, lying immediately anterior to the hip joint, and inserts directly on the lesser trochanter (**Fig. 2**).[9]

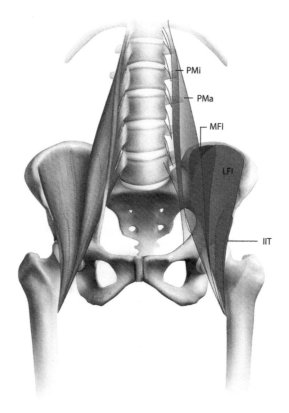

Fig. 1. AP anatomy of the iliopsoas musculotendinous unit as described by Tatu and colleagues[9] and Guillin and colleagues.[8] IIT, ilio-infratrochanteric muscle; LFI, lateral fibers of the iliacus; MFI, medial fibers of the iliacus; PMa, psoas major; PMi, psoas minor.

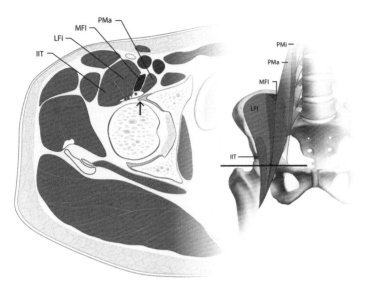

Fig. 2. Cross-sectional anatomy of the iliopsoas through the hip joint as described by Tatu and colleagues[9] and Guillin and colleagues.[8] The plane (*black line*) is demonstrated on the AP image. At this level, the iliacus (*double asterisk*) and psoas (*asterisk*) tendons are posterior to the iliopsoas muscle bundles and anterior to the hip joint and labrum (*arrow*).

Significant anatomic variability of the iliopsoas musculotendinous unit has been reported in the literature.[6,9–12] In a cadaveric study, Tatu and colleagues[9] reported the presence of 2 tendinous structures: the psoas major and iliacus tendons. The medial iliacus muscle bundle was shown to insert onto the iliacus tendon, which progressively converges with the larger and more medial psoas major tendon.[9] The lateral muscle bundle of the iliacus courses distally, without any tendinous attachments, and inserts on the anterior surface of the lesser trochanter and infratrochanteric ridge.[9] These findings were corroborated in a study by Guillin and colleagues[8] using ultrasound (US) to map the iliopsoas anatomy. Conversely, in a study using MRI with cadaveric correlation, Polster and coworkers[10] noted the medial iliacus bundle merged directly into the psoas major tendon, whereas the medial-most fibers of the lateral iliacus bundle inserted on a distinct thin intramuscular tendon. Philippon and colleagues[6] examined 53 fresh frozen cadavers and demonstrated at the level of the hip joint the prevalence of a single-, double-, and triple-banded iliopsoas tendon was noted 28.3%, 64.2%, and 7.5% of the time, respectively. In the pediatric population, the presence of 2 distinct tendons was observed in 21% of patients undergoing MRI.[11] Although controversy exists regarding the number of tendons and the relative contributions of the different muscle fibers to each tendon, the current literature challenges historical descriptions of a single common conjoint tendon.

The iliopsoas bursa, also known as the iliopectineal bursa, is positioned between the musculotendinous unit and the bony surfaces of the pelvis and proximal femur. It has been shown to be the largest bursa in the human body, typically extending from the iliopectineal eminence to the lower portion of the femoral head, with an average length of 5 to 6 cm and width of 3 cm.[9] Reports of communication of the bursa with the hip joint, through a congenital defect between the iliofemoral and pubofemoral ligaments, are variable. Tatu and colleagues[9] reported no communication in 14 cadaveric dissections; however, others have observed a direct communication between the joint and bursa in 15% of patients.[13] It is important to consider this communication during diagnostic injections, because the anesthetic material can move between the intra-articular and bursal compartments, confounding the results of the test.

The iliopsoas unit functions primarily as a powerful hip flexor, but also has important function in femoral external rotation and with lateral bending, flexion, and balance of the trunk.[14–17] The iliacus and psoas major have been shown to have individual and task-specific activation patterns.[14,16] The iliacus is important for stabilizing the pelvis[16] and for early rapid hip flexion while running.[14] The psoas major is important for sitting in an erect position and stability of the spine in the frontal plane.[16] Variable contribution of each muscle is observed during sit-ups depending on the angle of hip flexion.[16]

The psoas minor is a long slender muscle that originates from the vertebral bodies of T12 and L1 and is only present in 60% to 65% of individuals.[18,19] Distally, it merges with the iliac fascia and psoas major tendon, and in 90% of specimens, it has a firm bony attachment to the iliopectineal eminence.[19] The attachment to both the iliac fascia and the bony pelvis may assist in partially controlling the position and mechanical stability of the underlying iliopsoas as it crosses the femoral head.[19]

ILIOPSOAS SNAPPING

Iliopsoas snapping, also known as coxa saltans interna or internal hip snapping, is a disorder characterized by painful audible or palpable snapping of the iliopsoas during hip movement. Symptomatic snapping most commonly occurs with activities or sports that require significant hip range-of-motion, such as dance, soccer, hockey, and football,[20,21] and is observed more commonly in girls and women than in boys and men.[22] A history of acute trauma has been associated with the development of snapping in up to 50% of cases.[23] Although the true prevalence of this disorder is unknown, symptomatic snapping has been observed in up to 58% of elite ballet dancers.[21] Even so, the prevalence of asymptomatic snapping in the general population has been shown to be as high as 40%.[8] Therefore, careful assessment is important to determine if the snapping is symptomatic before proceeding with a treatment plan.

Snapping Mechanism

In 1951, Nunziata and Blumenfeld[24] first described the mechanism of internal coxa saltans as snapping of the iliopsoas tendon over the iliopectineal eminence of the pelvis. Since then, dynamic US has been used in several studies to confirm this mechanism as the primary source of iliopsoas snapping.[21,23,25–27] Most studies report a sudden "jerky" movement and audible or palpable snap of the iliopsoas over the iliopectineal eminence as the hip is brought from a position of flexion, abduction, and external rotation (FABER) to extension and neutral.

Although abnormal movement of the tendon over the iliopectineal eminence is commonly described as the source of the snapping phenomena, alternative mechanisms have been proposed. Several studies propose that soft tissue abnormalities, such as an accessory iliopsoas tendinous slip,[28] a paralabral cyst,[28] and/or stenosing tenosynovitis, are the source of snapping.[29] Other investigators have determined the iliopsoas snapping occurs over a bony prominence other than the iliopectineal eminence, such as the lesser trochanter[13] or the femoral head.[30] More recently, dynamic US has been used to demonstrate a sudden flipping of the psoas tendon over the iliacus muscle as the source of snapping.[8,21,28] In these studies, as the hip was flexed, abducted, and externally rotated, the iliacus became interposed between the psoas tendon and the superior pubic rami. As the hip was brought to neutral, part of the medial iliacus muscle became trapped as the tendon followed a reverse path to its original position. The trapped iliacus is suddenly released, resulting in an audible snap of the tendon against the pubic bone. Contrary to the original mechanism described by Nunziata and Blumenfeld, the iliopectineal eminence was medial to the psoas tendon and not involved with the observed snapping phenomena.[28] Overall, the exact mechanism of snapping remains controversial, and the lack of consensus regarding the mechanism supports the possibility of several potential causes for iliopsoas snapping.

Iliopsoas Bursitis and Tendonitis

Iliopsoas bursitis and tendonitis have been shown to be closely associated with the repetitive pathologic movement of the tendon observed in symptomatic coxa saltans interna.[13,26,31,32] The irregular movement of the tendon during the snapping phenomena is thought to cause irritation and inflammation of the underlying bursa.[33–35] Even so, some studies demonstrate no objective abnormality of the bursa in patients undergoing open surgery for symptomatic snapping.[13,36] Nevertheless, these conditions coexist so frequently that Johnston and coworkers[31] suggested they be considered a single entity referred to as "iliopsoas syndrome." Correspondingly, the diagnostic workup and treatment for these conditions are the same.

History and Physical Examination

The diagnosis of iliopsoas snapping begins with a thorough history. Patients often report painful snapping with hip movement during sporting or recreational activities. Patients may also have pre-existing asymptomatic snapping that becomes painful after repetitive training activities involving high hip flexion angles.[20] Symptoms can also occur during activities of daily living such as climbing stairs or standing from a sitting position.[37] The snapping sensation is accompanied by groin pain that may radiate into the thigh or top of the knee.

Physical examination should include a complete musculoskeletal evaluation of the hip and focused specialty tests specific for the suspected diagnosis. The most commonly described examination maneuver for detecting internal hip snapping is what is referred to as the "active iliopsoas snapping test." This test is performed by having the patient actively move the hip from the FABER position to extension and neutral (**Fig. 3**). The examiner's hand should be placed on the groin to palpate the iliopsoas snapping, which typically occurs with the hip at between 30° and 45° of flexion.[38] Iliopsoas strength is assessed by resisted hip flexion with the patient in the sitting position. Testing in this manner may also result in groin pain, but does not usually recreate snapping. Localized swelling of the inguinal region has been reported in up to 59% of patients with painful internal snapping.[26]

It is paramount to also evaluate the patient for external snapping of the iliotibial band (ITB) over the greater trochanter, which may present in a similar manner to iliopsoas snapping. Patients often report a sensation of the hip dislocating during the snapping event. The examination is the most efficient way to distinguish between internal and external hip snapping. The author's preferred examination technique, the "bicycle test," for determining the presence of external hip snapping is performed by having the patient actively cycle the affected extremity from flexion to extension while lying in the lateral decubitus position (**Fig. 4**). A palpable snap or clunk over the greater trochanter is confirmatory for this diagnosis.

Imaging

Although iliopsoas snapping is typically diagnosed with a thorough history and physical examination, imaging studies can be valuable for confirming the diagnosis and

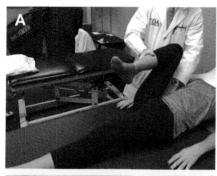
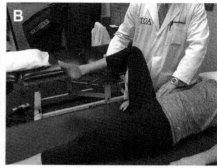
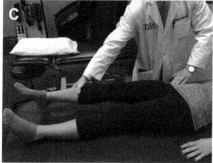

Fig. 3. The "active iliopsoas snapping test" for internal snapping of the iliopsoas. The patient actively moves the hip from flexion (*A*) to abduction and external rotation (*B*), and then to extension and neutral (*C*). A palpable clunk or pop is often felt with the examiner's hand placed over the hip.

identifying concomitant hip abnormality. Radiographic evaluation should begin with anteroposterior (AP) pelvis and lateral hip radiographs to rule out acute or chronic osseous abnormalities and to evaluate for radiographic signs of femoroacetabular impingement (FAI). In cases wherein the source of snapping is uncertain, dynamic US can be used to visualize the iliopsoas tendon or ITB during provocative maneuvers, such as the active iliopsoas snapping and bicycle tests.[8,21,23,25–28,32] US is also useful in identifying joint effusions and synovitis, rectus femoris tendinopathy, and iliopsoas bursitis and tendonitis.[26,32] In addition to also being able to detect iliopsoas tendinitis and bursitis,[23] MRI is useful in diagnosing associated chondral and labral abnormality, which are present in 67% to 100% of patients presenting with painful iliopsoas

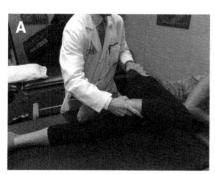
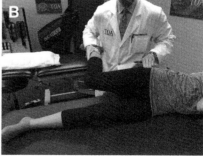

Fig. 4. The "bicycle test" for external snapping of the ITB. In the lateral decubitus position, the patient actively flexes (*A*) and then extends (*B*) the hip. A palpable, audible, and/or visible clunk can be detected over the greater trochanter.

snapping.[39–42] MRI can also determine the pathologic reason for snapping in up to 100% of patients.[26] In addition to formal imaging, US-guided injections of the iliopsoas bursa are useful in the evaluation of iliopsoas snapping (**Fig. 5**).[43] A preinjection and postinjection examination can be performed to determine if the patient experiences pain relief, and if so, supports the diagnosis of painful snapping.[39]

Surgical Treatment

Surgical treatment is considered in patients that have failed at least 3 months of a dedicated conservative program, including activity modification, physical therapy, nonsteroidal anti-inflammatory drugs (NSAIDs), and corticosteroid injections. The goal of surgical treatment is to lengthen the iliopsoas musculotendinous unit to prevent snapping and mechanical overpressurization of the underlying bursa.

Various techniques have been developed to release or lengthen the iliopsoas tendon. Historically, open surgery has been used; however, these procedures have increased morbidity and inferior results compared with arthroscopic techniques. In a systematic review of 11 studies, Khan and colleagues[44] demonstrated a complication rate of 21% in open procedures compared with 2.3% using arthroscopic techniques. Furthermore, patients undergoing open procedures had more postoperative pain, and recurrent snapping occurred in 23% of open compared with 0% of the arthroscopic surgeries.[44] In addition to lower complications and recurrent snapping, the arthroscopic approach can be used to diagnose and treat concomitant intra-articular abnormality. Treatment of associated intra-articular abnormalities in conjunction with iliopsoas snapping may result in improved patient-reported outcomes (PROs) relative to open procedures. Currently, however, there are no direct comparative studies evaluating open versus arthroscopic techniques for iliopsoas lengthening.

Arthroscopic release of the iliopsoas tendon has been described at 3 locations (**Fig. 6**): in the central compartment (**Fig. 7**),[40,41,45,46] in the peripheral compartment

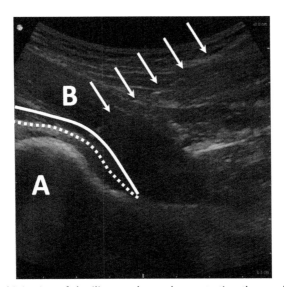

Fig. 5. US-guided injection of the iliopsoas bursa demonstrating the needle trajectory (*arrows*) toward the femoral head (*A*). The tip of the needle should penetrate through the iliopsoas muscle (*B*) into the iliopsoas bursa, which is located between the posterior surface of the iliopsoas (*solid line*) and the joint capsule (*dashed line*).

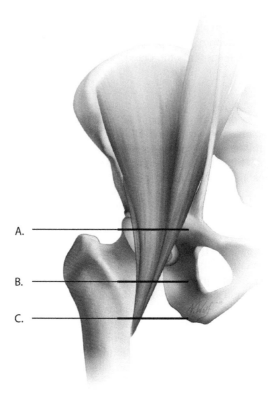

Fig. 6. The 3 described levels of iliopsoas release: central compartment (*A*), peripheral compartment (*B*), and lesser trochanter (*C*). At these levels, the ratio of tendon to muscle is 40% tendon/60% muscle belly, 53% tendon/47% muscle belly, and 60% tendon/40% muscle belly, respectively.

(**Fig. 8**),[47,48] and at the lesser trochanter (**Fig. 9**).[39,42,49,50] Level IV case series studies evaluating these techniques universally report good/excellent PROs, low recurrence rates, and minimal complications.[39–42,45–48] In a study evaluating athletes with painful iliopsoas snapping, Anderson and Keene[39] reported return to sport in all patients at an average of 9 months after release of the tendon at the lesser trochanter. In a level I randomized trial and a level IV comparative study, Ilizaliturri and colleagues[51,52] found favorable results with iliopsoas release either at the lesser trochanter or in the central compartment, with no significant differences between the techniques.

Although outcomes are generally good, transient weakness[39,41,42,47,48,50,52] and atrophy of the iliopsoas on MRI[53] have been observed after tenotomy. Even so, complete resolution of the weakness typically occurs by 3 to 6 months after surgery,[39,41,42] and no significant differences in hip flexion strength have been observed with tendon release at the different described levels.[44,51,52] The latter observation can partly be explained by the similar ratio of muscle to tendon volume observed at these locations.[54] Consequently, each technique results in a comparable volume of muscle fibers remaining intact within the musculotendinous unit, allowing similar forces to be generated for hip flexion.

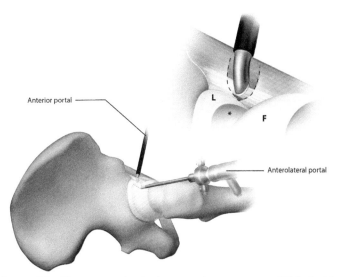

Fig. 7. Release of the iliopsoas tendon in the central compartment. With the hip under traction, a 70° arthroscope is placed in the anterolateral portal for visualization, and a beaver blade is used to extend the interportal capsulotomy medially (*dashed line*) to expose the iliopsoas tendon, located just anterior to the iliopsoas notch at the 3 o'clock position on the acetabulum (*asterisk*). The tendon can then be released with the blade or an electrocautery device, taking care to leave the muscular portion of iliopsoas intact, resulting in a fractional lengthening of the musculotendinous unit. F, femoral head; L, labrum.

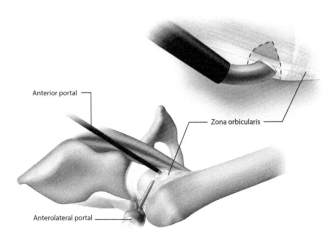

Fig. 8. Iliopsoas tenotomy in the peripheral compartment. To facilitate visualization, traction is released and the hip is placed in 30° of flexion. A 30° arthroscope is placed in the anterolateral portal and pointed anteriorly toward the joint capsule. The iliopsoas tendon can be identified through a small (1 cm) transverse capsulotomy (*dashed line*) lateral to the medial synovial fold and just proximal to the zona orbicularis anteriorly. An electrocautery device or beaver blade can then be used to divide the tendon.

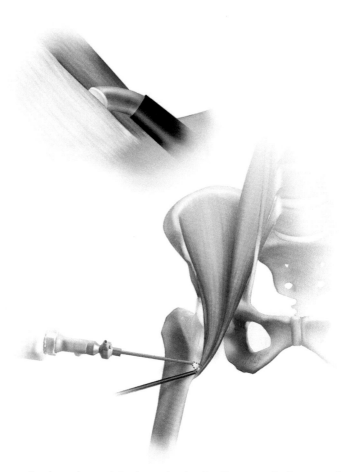

Fig. 9. Iliopsoas tendon release at the lesser trochanter. To access the lesser trochanter, the hip is flexed 30° and externally rotated until the lesser trochanter is parallel to the coronal plane of the body and maximally visualized with fluoroscopy. A spinal needle is then advanced anterior and perpendicular to the femur until it reaches the lesser trochanter. A cannula is placed in this position, and a second portal is made in a similar manner 5 to 7 cm distal to the first one. The 30° arthroscope is then placed in the proximal portal and electrocautery is used in the distal portal to clear any soft tissues and release the iliopsoas tendon at its insertion on the lesser trochanter.

Further studies have evaluated variables that are predictors of worse clinical outcomes.[40,46] In a level IV case series by Bitar and coworkers,[40] patients with recurrent snapping (18%) after iliopsoas lengthening in the central compartment had no improvements in PROs and had lower satisfaction and worse outcomes compared with those with resolution of snapping. In a separate level IV case series, Fabricant and colleagues[46] studied 67 consecutive patients undergoing iliopsoas release in the central compartment and determined patients with high femoral anteversion (>25°) had lower modified Harris hip scores (HHS) compared with patients that had normal to low (≤25°) femoral anteversion. They hypothesized that the iliopsoas may act as an important dynamic stabilizer given its anatomic location at the anterior aspect of the hip joint.[46] Overall, additional research is necessary to determine the best technique of iliopsoas release and further predictors of functional outcome and PROs.

ILIOPSOAS IMPINGEMENT

First described by Heyworth and colleagues[55] in 2007, iliopsoas impingement (IPI) is a pathomechanical process whereby an excessively tight iliopsoas tendon impinges on the underlying acetabular labrum, resulting in characteristic labral abnormality at the location of the psoas tendon on the acetabular rim. In this initial report, the investigators noted IPI and corresponding labral injury in 7 of 24 revision hip arthroscopy cases.[55] In each case, after iliopsoas release at the level of the acetabulum, the tendon no longer impinged on the anterior labrum during hip extension.[55] In a follow-up study at the same institution, Domb and coworkers[56] further defined the pathophysiologic mechanism of this phenomenon. In this study, the investigators identified 25 patients with direct anterior labral tears at the 3 o'clock position (right hip) in the absence of bony abnormalities. The location of labral abnormality corresponded to the iliopsoas notch (**Fig. 10**), directly beneath the iliopsoas tendon, which significantly differs from the traditional 1 to 2 o'clock location observed in FAI.[57,58] In some cases, the labrum appeared inflamed without frank tearing, which was referred to as the "IPI sign." Furthermore, adjacent tendinous inflammation and scarring of the tendon to the anterior capsule were observed in some patients. The investigators concluded that the labral injury was possibly the result of a tight iliopsoas impinging on the anterior labrum or a repetitive traction injury to the labrum from adherence of the tendon to the adjacent capsulolabral complex. Similar to the observations of Heyworth and colleagues, Domb and coworkers found releasing the tendon decreased compression on the underlying labrum in all cases. A cadaveric study by Yoshio and colleagues[59] demonstrated maximal pressure underneath the iliopsoas tendon occurs at the joint level during hip extension, supporting the possibility that excessive pathologic forces from the iliopsoas possibly results in labral injury.

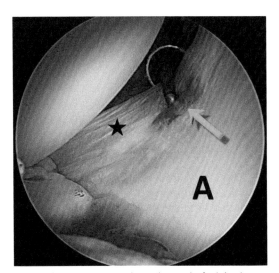

Fig. 10. Arthroscopic view from the posterolateral portal of a labral tear at the 3 o'clock position (*arrow*) in a patient with IPI. The iliopsoas notch, anterior labrum (*star*), and anterior acetabulum (*A*) are well visualized from this portal.

Iliopsoas impingement occurs most frequently in young active women, many who participate in regular sports.[45,56,60,61] Patients typically present with anterior groin pain that worsens with athletic activities and activities of daily living, such as active hip flexion, prolonged sitting, and getting out of a car.[45,56,60] Iliopsoas snapping is less commonly observed in IPI but has been reported in up to 17% of cases.[45,60] On physical examination, patients typically have a positive impingement test (flexion, adduction, and internal rotation), scour sign (flexion, adduction, and axial compression), and tenderness with manual compression over the iliopsoas.[45,56,60] Approximately half of the patients have pain with FABER and resisted straight leg-raise testing.[45,60] Intra-articular injections have shown variable results with some studies reporting transient improvement in 50% of patients,[56] whereas other studies report improved symptoms in all patients undergoing injection.[60] Plain film radiographs may show signs of FAI[45]; however, the most pertinent radiographic finding is a labral tear at or near the 3 o'clock position seen on MRI.[60]

Surgical management of IPI focuses on lengthening of the iliopsoas tendon and treatment of concurrent labral abnormality. Several studies have demonstrated favorable results with this treatment plan.[45,56,61] In the study by Domb and colleagues,[56] at an average of 21 months after arthroscopic tendon lengthening and either labral debridement or repair, 95% of patients surveyed reported their physical ability as "much improved" and none reported worse symptoms. HHS and hip outcome scores were available in 8 patients at final follow-up and demonstrated significant improvements compared with preoperative scores. Cascio and colleagues[61] reported on 16 hips with a minimum of 6-months follow-up that underwent tendon lengthening, with or without labral repair. The investigators noted the HHS improved from a mean of 70 preoperatively to 94 postoperatively; however, one patient required revision surgery at 18 months for repair of a labral tear that was not addressed at the initial surgery. Nelson and Keene[45] reported good to excellent results (modified HHS ≥80 points) in 23 of 30 patients undergoing tendon release for IPI. Patients with lower final PROs had avascular necrosis (n = 1), progressive degenerative joint disease (n = 1), trochanteric bursitis (n = 2), or recurrent painful iliopsoas snapping (n = 3). Two of the 3 patients with recurrent symptomatic snapping underwent a second iliopsoas release at the lesser trochanter and subsequently demonstrated good to excellent outcomes 1 year after the revision surgery. Although these level IV reports are encouraging, further studies with long-term follow-up are necessary to determine optimal treatment for IPI.

SUMMARY

The iliopsoas is an anatomically complex musculotendinous unit that functions primarily as a powerful hip flexor and secondarily as a femoral rotator and stabilizer of the lumbar spine and pelvis. Commonly described pathologic conditions of the involved the tendon-muscle complex include iliopsoas bursitis, tendonitis, impingement, and snapping. Initial treatment of iliopsoas disorders generally consists of a combination of physical therapy, activity modification, NSAIDs, and corticosteroid injections. If conservative treatment fails, arthroscopic surgery to address the existing pathologic condition has demonstrated encouraging results in mostly level IV studies. Further studies with a higher level of evidence and longer follow-up are needed to determine optimal treatments for these conditions.

REFERENCES

1. Serner A, Tol JL, Jomaah N, et al. Diagnosis of acute groin injuries: a prospective study of 110 athletes. Am J Sports Med 2015;43(8):1857–64.

2. Holmich P, Renstrom PA. Long-standing groin pain in sportspeople falls into three primary patterns, a "clinical entity" approach: a prospective study of 207 patients. Br J Sports Med 2007;41(4):247–52.
3. Holmich P, Thorborg K, Dehlendorff C, et al. Incidence and clinical presentation of groin injuries in sub-elite male soccer. Br J Sports Med 2014;48(16):1245–50.
4. Rankin AT, Bleakley CM, Cullen M. Hip joint pathology as a leading cause of groin pain in the sporting population: a 6-year review of 894 cases. Am J Sports Med 2015;43(7):1698–703.
5. Moore KL, Dalley AF. Clinically oriented anatomy. 4th edition. Baltimore (MD): Lippincott Williams & Wilkins; 1999. p. 533.
6. Philippon MJ, Devitt BM, Campbell KJ, et al. Anatomic variance of the iliopsoas tendon. Am J Sports Med 2014;42(4):807–11.
7. Lee K, Rosas H, Phancao JP. Snapping hip: imaging and treatment. Semin Musculoskelet Radiol 2013;17(03):286–94.
8. Guillin R, Cardinal É, Bureau NJ. Sonographic anatomy and dynamic study of the normal iliopsoas musculotendinous junction. Eur Radiol 2008;19(4):995–1001.
9. Tatu L, Parratte B, Vuillier F, et al. Descriptive anatomy of the femoral portion of the iliopsoas muscle. Anatomical basis of anterior snapping of the hip. Surg Radiol Anat 2001;23(6):371–4.
10. Polster JM, Elgabaly M, Lee H, et al. MRI and gross anatomy of the iliopsoas tendon complex. Skeletal Radiol 2007;37(1):55–8.
11. Crompton T, Lloyd C, Kokkinakis M, et al. The prevalence of bifid iliopsoas tendon on MRI in children. J Child Orthop 2014;8(4):333–6.
12. Shu B, Safran MR. Case report: bifid iliopsoas tendon causing refractory internal snapping hip. Clin Orthop Relat Res 2010;469(1):289–93.
13. Schaberg JE, Harper MC, Allen WC. The snapping hip syndrome. Am J Sports Med 1984;12(5):361–5.
14. Mann RA, Moran GT, Dougherty SE. Comparative electromyography of the lower extremity in jogging, running, and sprinting. Am J Sports Med 1986;14(6):501–10.
15. Fitzgerald P. The action of the iliopsoas muscle. Ir J Med Sci 1969;8(1):31–3.
16. Andersson E, Oddsson I , Grundström H, et al. The role of the psoas and iliacus muscles for stability and movement of the lumbar spine, pelvis and hip. Scand J Med Sci Sports 1995;5(1):10–6.
17. Rajendran K. The insertion of the iliopsoas as a design favouring lateral rather than medial rotation at the hip joint. Singapore Med J 1989;30(5):451–2.
18. Clemente CD. Anatomy: a regional atlas of the human body. 4th edition. Baltimore (MD): Lippincott Williams & Wilkins; 1997. p. 363.
19. Neumann DA, Garceau LR. A proposed novel function of the psoas minor revealed through cadaver dissection. Clin Anat 2014;28(2):243–52.
20. Wahl CJ, Warren RF, Adler RS, et al. Internal coxa saltans (snapping hip) as a result of overtraining: a report of 3 cases in professional athletes with a review of causes and the role of ultrasound in early diagnosis and management. Am J Sports Med 2004;32(5):1302–9.
21. Winston P, Awan R, Cassidy JD, et al. Clinical examination and ultrasound of self-reported snapping hip syndrome in elite ballet dancers. Am J Sports Med 2006;35(1):118–26.
22. Kroger E, Griesser M, Kolovich G, et al. Efficacy of surgery for internal snapping hip. Int J Sports Med 2013;34(10):851–5.
23. Janzen DL, Partridge E, Logan PM, et al. The snapping hip: clinical and imaging findings in transient subluxation of the iliopsoas tendon. Can Assoc Radiol J 1996;47(3):202–8.

24. Nunziata A, Blumenfeld I. Cadera a resorte: a proposito de una variedad. Prensa Med Argent 1951;38(32):1997–2001.

25. Cardinal E, Buckwalter KA, Capello WN, et al. US of the snapping iliopsoas tendon. Radiology 1996;198(2):521–2.

26. Wunderbaldinger P, Bremer C, Matuszewski L, et al. Efficient radiological assessment of the internal snapping hip syndrome. Eur Radiol 2001;11(9):1743–7.

27. Hashimoto BE, Green TM, Wiitala L. Ultrasonographic diagnosis of hip snapping related to iliopsoas tendon. J Ultrasound Med 1997;16(6):433–5.

28. Deslandes M, Guillin R, Cardinal E. The snapping iliopsoas tendon: new mechanisms using dynamic sonography. AJR Am J Roentgenol 2008;190(3):576–81.

29. Micheli LJ. Overuse injuries in children's sports: the growth factor. Orthop Clin North Am 1983;14(2):337–60.

30. Howse AJ. Orthopaedists aid ballet. Clin Orthop Relat Res 1972;89:52–63.

31. Johnston CA, Wiley JP, Lindsay DM, et al. Iliopsoas bursitis and tendinitis. A review. Sports Med 1998;25(4):271–83.

32. Pelsser V, Cardinal E, Hobden R, et al. Extraarticular snapping hip: sonographic findings. AJR Am J Roentgenol 2001;176(1):67–73.

33. Staple TW. Arthrographic demonstration of iliopsoas bursa extension of the hip joint. Radiology 1972;102(3):515–6.

34. Penkava RR. Iliopsoas bursitis demonstrated by computed tomography. AJR Am J Roentgenol 1980;135(1):175–6.

35. Peters JC, Coleman BG, Turner ML. CT evaluation of enlarged Iliopsoas bursa. AJR Am J Roentgenol 1980;135(2):392–4.

36. Jacobson T, Allen WC. Surgical correction of the snapping iliopsoas tendon. Am J Sports Med 1990;18(5):470–4.

37. Ilizaliturri VM Jr, Camacho-Galindo J. Endoscopic treatment of snapping hips, iliotibial band, and iliopsoas tendon. Sports Med Arthrosc 2010;18(2):120–7.

38. Sammarco GJ. The dancer's hip. Clin Sports Med 1983;2(3):485–98.

39. Anderson SA, Keene JS. Results of arthroscopic iliopsoas tendon release in competitive and recreational athletes. Am J Sports Med 2008;36(12):2363–71.

40. Bitar El YF, Stake CE, Dunne KF, et al. Arthroscopic iliopsoas fractional lengthening for internal snapping of the hip: clinical outcomes with a minimum 2-year follow-up. Am J Sports Med 2014;42(7):1696–703.

41. Contreras ME, Dani WS, Endges WK, et al. Arthroscopic treatment of the snapping iliopsoas tendon through the central compartment of the hip: a pilot study. J Bone Joint Surg Br 2010;92(6):777–80.

42. Flanum ME, Keene JS, Blankenbaker DG, et al. Arthroscopic treatment of the painful "internal" snapping hip: results of a new endoscopic technique and imaging protocol. Am J Sports Med 2007;35(5):770–9.

43. Blankenbaker DG, De Smet AA, Keene JS. Sonography of the iliopsoas tendon and injection of the iliopsoas bursa for diagnosis and management of the painful snapping hip. Skeletal Radiol 2006;35(8):565–71.

44. Khan M, Adamich J, Simunovic N. Surgical management of internal snapping hip syndrome: a systematic review evaluating open and arthroscopic approaches. Arthroscopy 2013;29(5):942–8.

45. Nelson IR, Keene JS. Results of labral-level arthroscopic iliopsoas tenotomies for the treatment of labral impingement. Arthroscopy 2014;30(6):688–94.

46. Fabricant PD, Bedi A, La Torre De K, et al. Clinical outcomes after arthroscopic psoas lengthening: the effect of femoral version. Arthroscopy 2012;28(7):965–71.

47. Hwang D-S, Hwang J-M, Kim P-S, et al. Arthroscopic treatment of symptomatic internal snapping hip with combined pathologies. Clin Orthop Surg 2015;7(2): 158–63.

48. Wettstein M, Jung J, Dienst M. Arthroscopic psoas tenotomy. Arthroscopy 2006; 22(8):907.e1–4.

49. Byrd JWT. Evaluation and management of the snapping iliopsoas tendon. Instr Course Lect 2006;55:347–55.

50. Ilizaliturri VM Jr, Villalobos FE Jr, Chaidez PA, et al. Internal snapping hip syndrome: treatment by endoscopic release of the iliopsoas tendon. Arthroscopy 2005;21(11):1375–80.

51. Ilizaliturri VM Jr, Buganza-Tepole M, Olivos-Meza A, et al. Central compartment release versus lesser trochanter release of the iliopsoas tendon for the treatment of internal snapping hip: a comparative study. Arthroscopy 2014;30(7):790–5.

52. Ilizaliturri VM, Chaidez C, Villegas P, et al. Prospective randomized study of 2 different techniques for endoscopic iliopsoas tendon release in the treatment of internal snapping hip syndrome. Arthroscopy 2009;25(2):159–63.

53. Hain KS, Blankenbaker DG, De Smet AA, et al. MR appearance and clinical significance of changes in the hip muscles and iliopsoas tendon after arthroscopic iliopsoas tenotomy in symptomatic patients. HSS J 2013;9(3):236–41.

54. Blomberg JR, Zellner BS, Keene JS. Cross-sectional analysis of iliopsoas muscle-tendon units at the sites of arthroscopic tenotomies: an anatomic study. Am J Sports Med 2011;39(Suppl):58S–63S.

55. Heyworth BE, Shindle MK, Voos JE, et al. Radiologic and intraoperative findings in revision hip arthroscopy. Arthroscopy 2007;23(12):1295–302.

56. Domb BG, Shindle MK, McArthur B, et al. Iliopsoas impingement: a newly identified cause of labral pathology in the hip. HSS J 2011;7(2):145–50.

57. Seldes RM, Tan V, Hunt J, et al. Anatomy, histologic features, and vascularity of the adult acetabular labrum. Clin Orthop Relat Res 2001;382:232–40.

58. Blankenbaker DG, De Smet AA, Keene JS, et al. Classification and localization of acetabular labral tears. Skeletal Radiol 2007;36(5):391–7.

59. Yoshio M, Murakami G, Sato T, et al. The function of the psoas major muscle: passive kinetics and morphological studies using donated cadavers. J Orthop Sci 2002;7(2):199–207.

60. Blankenbaker DG, Tuite MJ, Keene JS, et al. Labral injuries due to iliopsoas impingement: can they be diagnosed on MR arthrography? AJR Am J Roentgenol 2012;199(4):894–900.

61. Cascio BM, King D, Yen Y-M. Psoas impingement causing labrum tear: a series from three tertiary hip arthroscopy centers. J La State Med Soc 2013;165(2): 88–93.

Hip Instability
Current Concepts and Treatment Options

Guillaume D. Dumont, MD

KEYWORDS

- Hip instability • Hip joint capsule • Acetabular dysplasia • Capsular plication
- Periacetabular osteotomy

KEY POINTS

- Hip instability can result from traumatic injury with dislocation or subluxation; atraumatic capsular laxity, structural bony abnormality such as acetabular dysplasia; and iatrogenic injury.
- Repair of the capsulotomy during hip arthroscopy can help prevent iatrogenic instability.
- Some patients with borderline hip instability can be treated with arthroscopic surgery with labral preservation and capsular plication.
- Periacetabular osteotomy is the treatment of choice for acetabular dysplasia.

RELEVANT ANATOMY

The bony architecture of the hip provides inherent stability to the joint. The hip is generally viewed as an inherently constrained joint given the high degree of bony congruity between the femoral head and acetabulum. The orientation of the acetabulum can influence the stability of the joint, with a retroverted acetabulum predisposing one to posterior instability, whereas the anteverted acetabulum may predispose to anterior instability. In similar fashion, femoral version may influence hip stability if it diverges from its typical mild anteversion. The severely anteverted femoral neck is more prone to anterior instability. An elevated femoral neck-shaft angle is also associated with hip instability.

Acetabular coverage of the femoral head has been quantified using various measures, including the lateral center edge (LCE) angle, the anterior LCE angle, acetabular inclination (Tonnis angle), and the acetabular index[1] (**Fig. 1**). The LCE angle is often used as an initial measure of acetabular coverage (**Fig. 2**). A value of 25° or greater is typically considered normal, and less than 25° represents acetabular dysplasia. Values between 20° and 25° have sometimes been classified as borderline acetabular dysplasia.

Disclosure Statement: The author has nothing to disclose.
Department of Orthopaedic Surgery, University of South Carolina School of Medicine, 2 Medical Park Road, Suite 404, Columbia, SC 29203, USA
E-mail address: gddumont@gmail.com

A   **B**

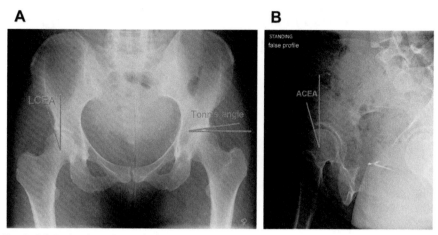

Fig. 1. (*A*) Evaluation of acetabular coverage starts with a well-rotated and tilted anteroposterior pelvis radiograph on which the LCE angle (LCEA) and Tonnis angle are measured. (*B*) Anterior center edge angle (ACEA) is measured on a false profile radiograph.

The iliofemoral, ischiofemoral, and pubofemoral ligaments make up the primary ligamentous static stabilizers of the hip.[2] In a cadaveric study, Martin and colleagues[3] quantified the contributions of each of these structures to external and internal rotation, through a range of flexion and extension of the hip. The iliofemoral ligament limits anterior translation of the femoral head and external rotation. Its lateral arm also contributed substantially to limiting internal rotation with the hip in extension. The pubofemoral ligament controls external rotation with the hip in extension, and the ischiofemoral ligament controls internal rotation with the hip in flexion or extension.

The acetabular labrum functions as a static stabilizer by deepening the hip socket and through the creation of a hydraulic fluid seal.[4,5] To evaluate the effect of a labral tearing on hip joint stability, Smith and colleagues[6] performed a cadaveric study in which nondysplastic hips were subjected to anterior femoral translational force,

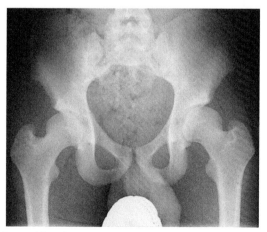

Fig. 2. Decreased femoral head coverage should raise concern for acetabular dysplasia and inherent hip instability.

comparing the intact labrum with radial tears of the labrum, 1-, 2-, and 3-cm circumferential tears of the labrum, 1-, 2-, and 3-cm partial labrectomy, and complete labrectomy. The investigators found that the acetabular labrum continues to function to resist femoral head translation despite circumferential chondrolabral separation. Radial tears decrease the strain of the adjacent acetabular labrum; however, removal of 2 cm or more of the labrum is was required to decrease gross stability of the hip. The findings of this study are helpful when considering the role of labral preservation versus labral debridement and may suggest that more aggressive labral debridement could potentially destabilize the hip, compared with repair of the torn acetabular labrum.

In a cadaveric study of 15 hips, anterior translation and external rotation were measured using implanted tantalum beads in hips with an intact labrum and iliofemoral ligament, sectioned labrum, and/or iliofemoral ligament and repaired the labrum and iliofemoral ligament. The iliofemoral ligament had a significant role in limiting external rotation and anterior translation of the femur. The acetabular labrum had a secondary stabilizing role in stabilizing these motions. Repair of the labrum and iliofemoral ligament did seem to restore range of motion to the nonsectioned state.[7]

TRAUMATIC INSTABILITY

Traumatic dislocation of the hip occurs with dislocation or subluxation of the hip secondary to an event such as motor vehicle crash, sports injury, or after iatrogenic injury. Most traumatic and athletic type dislocations are posterior, and are typically caused by a posteriorly directed force through the knee, with the knee and hip flexed. Associated fractures of the femur or acetabulum may be present (**Fig. 3**). Traumatic subluxation is subtler in its presentation and may be the result of a posteriorly directed force on the limb through a flex hip or a twisting motion or sudden change of direction. Sports-related traumatic instability of the hip is the result of relatively low-energy mechanisms compared with vehicular trauma.[8] Subluxation events of the hip are more frequently encountered than dislocations.[9] Anterior hip instability is less common than posterior instability and may be caused by an anteriorly directed force or contact on the externally rotated and extended hip. Anterior instability is often associated with dysplasia; supraphysiologic joint motion as required in sports, such as gymnastics, dance, and figure skating; or iatrogenic injury to the anterior hip capsule.[10,11]

MICROINSTABILITY AND THE IMPLICATION OF FEMOROACETABULAR IMPINGEMENT

The bony morphologic characteristics associated with femoroacetabular impingement (FAI) have been implicated with both traumatic and nontraumatic instability of the hip. A recent systematic noted that FAI morphologic characteristics may predispose the hip to instability through anatomic conflict of the pincer and/or cam lesions levering the femoral head posteriorly. The review included 4 clinical studies and 3 basic science studies. The clinical studies included a total of 92 patients. Eighty-nine out of 92 patients were found to have morphologic characteristics of FAI (74% cam; 64% pincer).[12]

One study by Charbonnier and colleagues[13] used MRI to perform 3-dimensional motion analysis of the hips of 11 professional dancers. Although none of the patients had radiologic characteristics of FAI, impingement was noted in 70% of hips with certain positions and subluxation was noted in 39% of hips. The average translation distance of the femoral head with deep hip flexion was 5 mm. All instances of subluxation were associated with impingement. Another MRI study by Kolo and colleagues[14] was inclusive of the patients in the prior study. Twenty-five dancers underwent MRI in

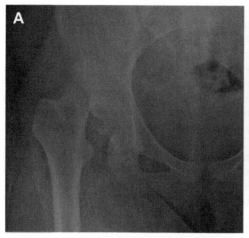
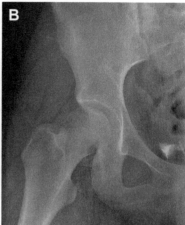
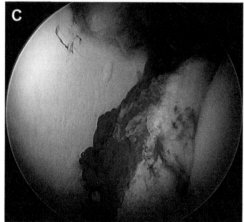

Fig. 3. Radiograph of a posterior hip dislocation (*A*) with residual joint space incongruity after closed reduction (*B*). A displaced posterior wall fracture and bucket-handle labral tear is identified during arthroscopy (*C*) blocking a congruent reduction.

the splits position, showing an average femoral head subluxation of 2.05 mm in this position. Wassilew and colleagues[15] used dynamic volume-rendered computed tomography (CT) to demonstrate anterior impingement and posterior subluxation with deep flexion and posterior impingement and anterior subluxation with abduction/external rotation of the hip.

Canham and colleagues[12] note that the mechanism by which FAI predisposes the hip to instability is likely multifactorial. The acetabular labrum adds depth to the acetabulum and is more often compromised in patients with FAI, thus potentially contributing to instability. Attenuation of the hip capsule and weakness of the dynamic stabilizers of the hip may also play a role.

DEVELOPMENTAL DYSPLASIA OF THE HIP

In developmental dysplasia of the hip, the morphologically abnormal acetabulum is too shallow and may result in instability of the joint. The decrease in bony acetabular coverage results in increased stress on the acetabular labrum. Gupta and colleagues[16] investigated labral size in a dysplastic hips compared with nondysplastic hips and found that the labrum was significantly larger in dysplastic hips. The mean difference in the width of the labrum was most substantial at the anterosuperior quadrant, where it was approximately 1.0 mm (5.6 mm vs 4.66 mm). This increase in labral size should not necessarily be relied on for diagnosis of instability. A study whereby the labrum was visualized in 553 patients undergoing hip preservation surgery noted that the labrum was characterized as hypertrophic in 50% of hips, normal in 45% of hips, hypoplastic in 4%, and ossified in 1%. Decreased LCE angle and anterior center edge angle, indicating more severe dysplasia, were associated with labral hypertrophy; however, chronicity of symptoms was not.[17]

IATROGENIC HIP INSTABILITY

The iliofemoral ligament is a primary stabilizing structure for controlling anterior translation and external rotation. It is incised during the commonly used interportal capsulotomy between the anterolateral portal and the anterior portal. In certain settings, this may contribute to instability of the hip (**Fig. 4**). Anterior and posterior dislocation of the hip has also been reported after hip arthroscopy.[18–23] Most surgeons using the T-capsulotomy advocate for routine closure of the capsulotomy, and many surgeons performing the less invasive interportal capsulotomy are routinely closing the capsulotomy.[24,25] Risk factors that should influence the surgeon to repair the capsulotomy include connective tissue disorders and supraphysiologic laxity as determined by physical examination maneuvers; activities involving supraphysiologic range of motion of the hip, including gymnastics, figure skating, ballet, and martial arts; large cam lesions leaving a capacious space after femoroplasty; increased femoral anteversion; acetabular dysplasia; and patients with a history of hip instability.[26,27]

EVALUATION
History

The athlete with a hip dislocation will typically be identified immediately based on substantial symptoms of pain and inability to bear weight. Those suffering a subluxation episode of the hip or with more subtle instability may not necessarily report overt

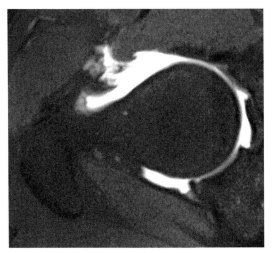

Fig. 4. Magnetic resonance arthrogram after a prior hip arthroscopy demonstrating a large defect in the anterior hip capsule. This defect may contribute to postoperative iatrogenic instability.

symptoms of hip laxity or giving way. Often the predominant presenting symptom is groin or anterolateral hip pain. In cases of posterior instability, posterior hip/buttock pain may be present. Symptoms may be modest, and the athlete may not be completely disabled from playing. Persistence of symptoms or worsening of symptoms should prompt more thorough evaluation.[10] Connective tissues disorders, such as Marfan syndrome and Ehlers-Danlos, may also present with symptoms of hip instability; an effort should be made to identify global symptoms of joint hypermobility.

Physical Examination

If patients are ambulatory, gait should be inspected initially to identify a limp. Initial observation of the posteriorly dislocated hip typically shows a flexed, internally rotated, adducted, and shortened limb. In the case of an anterior dislocation, the hip is usually externally rotated, extended, and abducted. Provocative maneuvers can elicit symptoms of pain or apprehension in patients who have suffered a subluxation or if more subtle instability is present. Axial loading of the flexed hip will elicit discomfort in cases of posterior instability, whereas abduction and external rotation will produce discomfort in cases of anterior instability.

Imaging

Plain radiographs including an anteroposterior view of the pelvis and a lateral view of the hip should be obtained initially to evaluate for concentric reduction of the hip joint and to assess for associated fractures or intra-articular bony fragments. CT is sometimes necessary to aid with the latter. The presence or absence and the pattern of associated fractures typically guides initial treatment, with pure dislocations often not requiring any further intervention. MRI of the hip is useful to evaluate for chondrolabral injury or bony edema/impaction of the femoral head or acetabulum. In the subacute setting, MRI may identify early signs of avascular necrosis.

TREATMENT
Nonoperative Treatment

Patients with dislocations of the hip should undergo emergent closed reduction of the hip to minimize the risk of avascular necrosis of the femoral head. Postreduction imaging is important to confirm concentric reduction and to ensure that no intra-articular bony fragments are present. Most patients with acute traumatic subluxations can be treated nonsurgically with a period of restricted weight bearing. Byrd and colleagues[10] recommend a period of 4 weeks of restricted weight bearing and an overall 3-month period to allow for acute symptoms to resolve and allow an opportunity for associated intra-articular structural injuries to declare themselves. A structured physical therapy program is engaged to gradually return the athlete to activities during this period. If symptoms persist 3 months after the injury, further investigative imaging is warranted to elucidate the cause. Return to play is reasonable after 8 to 10 weeks if symptoms have resolved.

Acute Surgical Treatment

Immediate surgery may be required if entrapped bony fragments are noted after reduction of a dislocated hip. Fragment removal may be performed through arthrotomy or arthroscopically. Associated pathology, including FAI and labral tear, may be noted; the surgeon may choose to address these findings during the same surgical setting if they are deemed to have been contributing to patients' symptoms.[28] Surgical treatment may also be required for a variety of femoral head or acetabular fracture patterns.

Arthroscopy in Patients with Dysplasia

Acetabular dysplasia has generally been viewed as a contraindication to hip arthroscopy. Cases of catastrophic dislocation after arthroscopy in the setting of acetabular dysplasia have been reported. Arthroscopic management cannot correct the underlying bony deficiency; thus, many dysplastic patients are better served with pelvic/acetabular osteotomy to address their bony deficiency. Byrd and Jones,[29] in 2003, suggested that the results of hip arthroscopy are influenced more so by the presence of and nature of intra-articular pathology and not simply by the absence or presence of dysplasia. In this study of dysplastic (LCE angle <20) and borderline dysplastic (LCE angle 20–25) patients undergoing hip arthroscopy with various interventions, improvements in the modified Harris Hip Score (mHHS) comparable with those in the nondysplastic population were noted. The investigators note, however, that hip arthroscopy should be considered just one tool in a complement of resources needed to assess and treat the dysplastic hip.[29]

Larson and colleagues[30] compared 88 hips with dysplasia with an age-matched cohort of 231 hips without radiographic evidence of dysplasia. The patients underwent labral repairs (76%), labral debridement (23%), capsular repair/plication (82%), and femoral osteochondroplasty (72%). The group of patients with acetabular dysplasia (mean LCE angle 20.8 and Tonnis angle 11.0) showed improvement in mHHS, though it was a less substantial improvement than seen in patients without dysplasia (Delta 15.6 vs 24.4). The dysplastic cohort had 60.9% good/excellent results compared with 81.2% in the nondysplastic group. Failure, defined as mHHS of 70 or less or subsequent femoral/pelvic osteotomy or total hip arthroplasty, was seen in 32.2% of dysplastic hips versus 10.5% of nondysplastic hips. Patients with dysplastic hips who underwent capsular plication with labral repair fared better than the remainder of patients with dysplastic hips.[30]

Fukui and colleagues[31] evaluated 80 hips with a lateral center edge angle of 20° to 25° treated with hip arthroscopy, labral repair, correction of femoroacetabular impingement, and capsular closure at a mean follow-up of 40 months. The mHHS improved from a mean of 63.5 to 84.9 points. The Western Ontario and McMaster Universities Arthritis Index and SF-12 Physical Component summary score also showed significant improvements. Revision hip arthroscopy was performed on 7 patients, and 5 patients required total hip arthroplasty. Jayasekera and colleagues[32] noted good pain relief at 1 year in patients with acetabular dysplasia treated with hip arthroscopy but did emphasize that this treatment does not address underlying acetabular bony abnormality.

Arthroscopic Capsular Plication

Patients with hip dysplasia are at an increased risk for instability after arthroscopic treatment, and the surgeon should be mindful to repair the capsulotomy. Techniques for capsular plication and inferior capsular shift have been described. The goal of this technique is to imbricate the capsule and create an inferior shift of the capsule to augment the screw-home mechanism of the iliofemoral ligament.[33,34]

Domb and colleagues[35] described their results with arthroscopic surgery in patients with borderline dysplasia (LCE angle 18–25). Twenty-two of their patients were available for follow-up, at a mean of 27.5 months. Intra-articular pathology was treated, and capsular plication with inferior shift was performed. The investigators reported significant improvement in all patient outcome scores. Two of their patients underwent revision hip arthroscopy.

In patients presenting with hip instability after hip arthroscopy without repair of the capsulotomy site, secondary repair may be helpful in restoring stability and reducing pain. Wylie and colleagues identified a cohort of 20 patients who underwent revision hip arthroscopy for repair of the interportal capsulotomy for symptomatic hip instability. The mean age of the patients was 29.7 years old. The mean LCE angle and acetabular index were 25° and 7°, respectively. This group of patients had limited improvement 19.1 months after the index procedure as shown on mHHS (57.1–57.6), Hip Outcome Score (HOS)–activities of daily living (ADL) (62.7–66.4), and HOS-Sports (42.0–39.1). One year after revision surgery (closure of the capsule), substantial improvement in functional scores was noted (mHHS 57.6–85.8; HOS-ADL 66.4–85.7; HOS-Sports 39.1–79.8). Similar results continued in the smaller portion of the cohort with the 2-year follow-up.[36]

In response to patients with continued symptoms after hip arthroscopy with capsulotomy (without capsular closure) or capsulectomy, capsular reconstruction using allograft iliotibial band has been described. The technique aims to decrease symptoms from microinstability or pain from invagination of overlying muscle into the capsular defect.[37] Future studies assessing patient outcomes after these techniques will be informative.

It is promising that arthroscopic management may result in improvement of certain subsets of hips with characteristics of instability. Nonetheless, a higher rate of failure remains in the dysplastic cohort; if the surgeon chooses to perform arthroscopic hip surgery in this setting, patients should be made aware of the potential failure to improve due to underlying bony coverage deficiency and the higher-than-normal likelihood that a secondary open operation might be necessary. In addition, it would seem that arthroscopic treatment of the dysplastic hip should include capsular repair/plication if a capsulotomy is performed.

Limitations of Arthroscopy

Given the mixed results noted in patients with varying degrees of acetabular dysplasia undergoing hip arthroscopy, diagnostic criteria are needed to aid in selecting those who may benefit from this treatment modality versus those who would be better served with alternate surgical options. Uchida and colleagues[38] examined clinical and radiographic predictors associated with worsened clinical outcomes in patients treated with hip arthroscopy, labral preservation, and capsular closure. The investigators found that the presence of a broken Shenton line, femoral neck-shaft angle greater than 140°, LCE angle less than 19°, body mass index greater than 23 kg/m^2, higher grades of acetabular cartilage damage, and femoral head cartilage damage were all predictive of poorer outcomes. Of these factors, the broken Shenton line and elevated femoral neck-shaft angle were most predictive of failure. Patients with these characteristics do not seem to be good candidates for arthroscopic management.[38]

Another study by Ross and colleagues[39] identified a cohort of patients who failed hip arthroscopy and ultimately underwent periacetabular osteotomy (PAO). They found that failed hip arthroscopy and the need for PAO were more commonly observed in young females with mild/moderate dysplasia, major functional limitations, and intra-articular abnormalities. In dysplastic patients treated with hip arthroscopy, those found to have chondral damage, especially to the anterior acetabulum and posterior femoral head, are more likely to require conversion to total hip arthrosplasty.[40] In a multicenter trial of the Academic Network of Conservation Hip Outcome Research (ANCHOR) group, the most common cause for revision hip preservation surgery was noted to be persistent structural disease. Secondary surgery included deformity correction with femoral osteochondroplasty and/or PAO.[41]

Recognition of dysplasia is requisite to guide appropriate treatment. The LCE angle is most widely used; however, Pereira and colleagues[42] suggest the measurement of this single variable may lead to underdiagnosis of acetabular dysplasia. The investigators recommend the addition of one adjunct measurement in patients with mild/borderline dysplasia and suggest the use of the Tonnis angle.

Periacetabular Osteotomy

The Bernese PAO provides a useful tool that allows for extensive reorientation of the acetabulum in the setting of dysplasia (**Fig. 5**). The procedure aims to reduce the long-term effects of altered joint biomechanics causing increased peak contact pressures and edge loading of the acetabular rim. The procedure involves 3 bony cuts in the ischium, pubis, and ilium.[43] Systematic review of outcomes after PAO have shown good pain relief and function at the short- to midterm follow-up.[44,45]

Concomitant Arthroscopy and Periacetabular Osteotomy

Although arthroscopy in isolation may not be indicated in some patients with dysplasia of the hip, it may be useful as an adjunct treatment in cases of concurrent dysplasia and FAI as well as for intraarticular pathology (**Fig. 6**). Although PAO is a reliable technique for correcting bony undercoverage of the acetabulum, arthroscopy is well suited for identification and treatment of intra-articular pathology. Ross and colleagues[46] examined the potential role of adjunct arthroscopy in patients undergoing PAO. These investigators found that 63% of patients who underwent PAO had a central compartment abnormality that was amenable to arthroscopic treatment. Those with more severe dysplasia (LCE angle <15° and acetabular inclination >20°) had more severe chondrolabral disease.

Domb and colleagues[47] describe their early outcomes with concomitant hip arthroscopy and PAO. Seventeen patients underwent hip arthroscopy for evaluation and treatment of intra-articular pathology and femoral osteochondroplasty, followed by PAO to correct acetabular coverage deficits. The LCE angle was improved from 11° to 29°. The anterior center edge angle increased from 7° preoperatively to 27° postoperatively, and the acetabular inclination angle decreased from 18° to 3°. In sum, these values represent correction of the structural bony pelvis/acetabular abnormality. An excellent outcome was obtained in 82% of patients. The additional of hip arthroscopy did not seem to introduce complications beyond those known and attributed to PAO.[47]

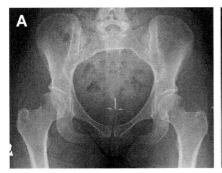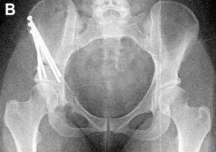

Fig. 5. (*A*) Anteroposterior pelvis demonstrating bilateral acetabular dysplasia. (*B*) Bernese-type PAO is effective for improving femoral head coverage and inherent hip stability in cases of acetabular dysplasia.

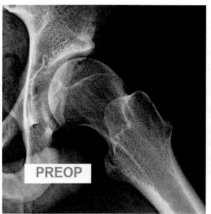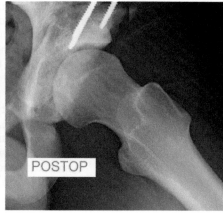

Fig. 6. In cases of concurrent impingement and acetabular dysplasia or when labral pathology has been identified, combined hip arthroscopy and PAO is useful to treat all contributory pathology. POSTOP, postoperative; PREOP, preoperative.

PAO after failed hip arthroscopy in patients with dysplasia seems to yield similar results to PAO performed as the index procedure. No difference in the risk of progression to total hip arthroplasty was identified in these two cohorts, in a study by Kain and colleagues.[48]

SUMMARY

Hip instability can present in a variety of ways ranging from acute traumatic dislocations and subluxations to chronic microinstability related to anatomic deficits, such as acetabular dysplasia and iatrogenic capsulotomy. It is important to carefully investigate the underlying cause of instability to make its accurate diagnosis. Emerging arthroscopic techniques have shown promising outcomes in treating certain anatomic abnormalities associated with instability, though limitations of these techniques must be respected. PAO remains the mainstay of treatment of structural correction of acetabular dysplasia.

REFERENCES

1. Clohisy JC, Carlisle JC, Beaule PE, et al. A systematic approach to the plain radiographic evaluation of the young adult hip. J Bone Joint Surg Am 2008; 90(Suppl 4):47–66.
2. Telleria JJ, Lindsey DP, Giori NJ, et al. An anatomic arthroscopic description of the hip capsular ligaments for the hip arthroscopist. Arthroscopy 2011;27: 628–36.
3. Martin HD, Savage A, Braly BA, et al. The function of the hip capsular ligaments: a quantitative report. Arthroscopy 2008;24:188–95.
4. Ferguson SJ, Bryant JT, Ganz R, et al. An in vitro investigation of the acetabular labral seal in hip joint mechanics. J Biomech 2003;36:171–8.
5. Ferguson SJ, Bryant JT, Ganz R, et al. The acetabular labrum seal: a poroelastic finite element model. Clin Biomech 2000;15:463–8.
6. Smith MV, Panchal HB, Ruberte Thiele RA, et al. Effect of acetabular labrum tears on hip stability and labral strain in a joint compression model. Am J Sports Med 2011;39(Suppl):103S–10S.

7. Myers CA, Register BC, Lertwanich P, et al. Role of the acetabular labrum and the iliofemoral ligament in hip stability: an in vitro biplane fluoroscopy study. Am J Sports Med 2011;39(Suppl):85S–91S.

8. Moorman CT 3rd, Warren RF, Hershman EB, et al. Traumatic posterior hip subluxation in American football. J Bone Joint Surg Am 2003;85-A:1190–6.

9. Foulk DM, Mullis BH. Hip dislocation: evaluation and management. J Am Acad Orthop Surg 2010;18:199–209.

10. Byrd JWT, Maiers II P. Traumatic instability: acute and delayed management. In: Nho SJ, editor. Hip arthroscopy and hip joint preservation surgery. New York: Springer; 2015. p. 961–70.

11. Shu B, Safran MR. Hip instability: anatomic and clinical considerations of traumatic and atraumatic instability. Clin Sports Med 2011;30:349–67.

12. Canham CD, Yen YM, Giordano BD. Does femoroacetabular impingement cause hip instability? A systematic review. Arthroscopy 2016;32(1):203–8.

13. Charbonnier C, Kolo FC, Duthon VB, et al. Assessment of congruence and impingement of the hip joint in professional ballet dancers: a motion capture study. Am J Sports Med 2011;39:557–66.

14. Kolo FC, Charbonnier C, Pfirrmann CW, et al. Extreme hip motion in professional ballet dancers: dynamic and morphological evaluation based on magnetic resonance imaging. Skeletal Radiol 2013;42:689–98.

15. Wassilew GI, Janz V, Heller MO, et al. Real time visualization of femoroacetabular impingement and subluxation using 320-slice computed tomography. J Orthop Res 2013;31:275–81.

16. Gupta A, Chandrasekaran S, Redmond JM, et al. Does labral size correlate with degree of acetabular dysplasia? Orthop J Sports Med 2015;3. 2325967115572573.

17. Sankar WN, Beaule PE, Clohisy JC, et al. Labral morphologic characteristics in patients with symptomatic acetabular dysplasia. Am J Sports Med 2015;43: 2152–6.

18. Rosenbaum A, Roberts T, Flaherty M, et al. Posterior dislocation of the hip following arthroscopy - a case report and discussion. Bull I Iosp Joint Dis 2014; 72:181–4.

19. Austin DC, Horneff JG 3rd, Kelly JD. Anterior hip dislocation 5 months after hip arthroscopy. Arthroscopy 2014;30:1380–2.

20. Matsuda DK. Acute iatrogenic dislocation following hip impingement arthroscopic surgery. Arthroscopy 2009;25:400–4.

21. Mei-Dan O, McConkey MO, Brick M. Catastrophic failure of hip arthroscopy due to iatrogenic instability: can partial division of the ligamentum teres and iliofemoral ligament cause subluxation? Arthroscopy 2012;28:440–5.

22. Ranawat AS, McClincy M, Sekiya JK. Anterior dislocation of the hip after arthroscopy in a patient with capsular laxity of the hip. A case report. J Bone Joint Surg Am 2009;91:192–7.

23. Sansone M, Ahlden M, Jonasson P, et al. Total dislocation of the hip joint after arthroscopy and ileopsoas tenotomy. Knee Surg Sports Traumatol Arthrosc 2013;21:420–3.

24. Frank RM, Lee S, Bush-Joseph CA, et al. Improved outcomes after hip arthroscopic surgery in patients undergoing T-capsulotomy with complete repair versus partial repair for femoroacetabular impingement: a comparative matched-pair analysis. Am J Sports Med 2014;42:2634–42.

25. Harris JD, Slikker W 3rd, Gupta AK, et al. Routine complete capsular closure during hip arthroscopy. Arthrosc Tech 2013;2:e89–94.

26. Nepple JJ, Smith MV. Biomechanics of the hip capsule and capsule management strategies in hip arthroscopy. Sports Med Arthrosc 2015;23:164–8.

27. Larson CM, Stone RM, Grossi EF, et al. Ehlers-Danlos syndrome: arthroscopic management for extreme soft-tissue hip instability. Arthroscopy 2015;31: 2287–94.

28. Philippon MJ, Kuppersmith DA, Wolff AB, et al. Arthroscopic findings following traumatic hip dislocation in 14 professional athletes. Arthroscopy 2009;25: 169–74.

29. Byrd JW, Jones KS. Hip arthroscopy in the presence of dysplasia. Arthroscopy 2003;19:1055–60.

30. Larson CM, Ross JR, Stone RM, et al. Arthroscopic management of dysplastic hip deformities: predictors of success and failures with comparison to an arthroscopic FAI cohort. Am J Sports Med 2016;44(2):447–53.

31. Fukui K, Trindade CA, Briggs KK, et al. Arthroscopy of the hip for patients with mild to moderate developmental dysplasia of the hip and femoroacetabular impingement: outcomes following hip arthroscopy for treatment of chondrolabral damage. Bone Joint J 2015;97-B:1316–21.

32. Jayasekera N, Aprato A, Villar RN. Hip arthroscopy in the presence of acetabular dysplasia. Open Orthop J 2015;9:185–7.

33. Chandrasekaran S, Vemula SP, Martin TJ, et al. Arthroscopic technique of capsular plication for the treatment of hip instability. Arthrosc Tech 2015;4: e163–7.

34. Smith MV, Sekiya JK. Hip instability. Sports Med Arthrosc 2010;18:108–12.

35. Domb BG, Stake CE, Lindner D, et al. Arthroscopic capsular plication and labral preservation in borderline hip dysplasia: two-year clinical outcomes of a surgical approach to a challenging problem. Am J Sports Med 2013;41:2591–8.

36. Wylie JD, Beckmann JT, Maak TG, et al. Arthroscopic capsular repair for symptomatic hip instability after previous hip arthroscopic surgery. Am J Sports Med 2016;44(1):39–45.

37. Trindade CA, Sawyer GA, Fukui K, et al. Arthroscopic capsule reconstruction in the hip using iliotibial band allograft. Arthrosc Tech 2015;4:e71–4.

38. Uchida S, Utsunomiya H, Mori T, et al. Clinical and radiographic predictors for worsened clinical outcomes after hip arthroscopic labral preservation and capsular closure in developmental dysplasia of the hip. Am J Sports Med 2016;44(1):28–38.

39. Ross JR, Clohisy JC, Baca G, et al. Patient and disease characteristics associated with hip arthroscopy failure in acetabular dysplasia. J Arthroplasty 2014; 29:160–3.

40. Dwyer MK, Lee JA, McCarthy JC. Cartilage status at time of arthroscopy predicts failure in patients with hip dysplasia. J Arthroplasty 2015;30:121–4.

41. Clohisy JC, Nepple JJ, Larson CM, et al, Academic Network of Conservation Hip Outcome Research (ANCHOR) Members. Persistent structural disease is the most common cause of repeat hip preservation surgery. Clin Orthop Relat Res 2013;471:3788–94.

42. Pereira F, Giles A, Wood G, et al. Recognition of minor adult hip dysplasia: which anatomical indices are important? Hip Int 2014;24:175–9.

43. Ganz R, Klaue K, Vinh TS, et al. A new periacetabular osteotomy for the treatment of hip dysplasias. Technique and preliminary results. Clin Orthop Relat Res 1988;(232):26–36.

44. Clohisy JC, Schutz AL, St John L, et al. Periacetabular osteotomy: a systematic literature review. Clin Orthop Relat Res 2009;467:2041–52.

45. Lodhia P, Chandrasekaran S, Gui C, et al. Open and arthroscopic treatment of adult hip dysplasia: a systematic review. Arthroscopy 2016;32(2):374–83.
46. Ross JR, Zaltz I, Nepple JJ, et al. Arthroscopic disease classification and interventions as an adjunct in the treatment of acetabular dysplasia. Am J Sports Med 2011;39(Suppl):72S–8S.
47. Domb BG, LaReau JM, Hammarstedt JE, et al. Concomitant hip arthroscopy and periacetabular osteotomy. Arthroscopy 2015;31:2199–206.
48. Kain MS, Novais EN, Vallim C, et al. Periacetabular osteotomy after failed hip arthroscopy for labral tears in patients with acetabular dysplasia. J Bone Joint Surg Am 2011;93(Suppl 2):57–61.

Peritrochanteric Endoscopy

Brian A. Mosier, MD, Noah J. Quinlan, MD, Scott D. Martin, MD*

KEYWORDS

- Gluteal tears • Coxa saltans • Trochanteric bursitis

KEY POINTS

- Most peritrochanteric disorders can be effectively treated with conservative nonoperative therapies.
- Tears of the gluteus medius and minimus tendons can be reliably repaired using endoscopic techniques with an excellent return of function.
- As understanding of peritrochanteric disorders improves, the indication for endoscopic intervention will be expanded.

 Video content accompanies this article at http://www.sportsmed.theclinics.com.

INTRODUCTION

Lateral-sided hip pain can present a daunting treatment challenge; however, with accurate diagnosis and appropriate intervention patients can experience remarkable improvements in pain and function. As our knowledge of the complex anatomical relationships and intricate structural dynamics of the peritrochanteric space improve, we are better able to accurately assess this patient population. With recent technological advancements in intracapsular arthroscopy, these tools are being increasingly applied to endoscopy of the peritrochanteric space with good outcomes.[1–4] This article focuses on the current indications and techniques for endoscopic repair of peritrochanteric hip disorders.

GLUTEUS MEDIUS AND MINIMUS TEARS

The first descriptions of gluteal tendon tears occurred in the late 1990s when they were described as incidental findings during surgical treatment for femoral neck fractures

Disclosure Statement: The authors have nothing to disclose.
Orthopedic Surgery, Brigham and Women's Hospital/Harvard Medical School, 75 Francis Street, Boston, MA 02115, USA
* Corresponding author.
E-mail address: sdmartin@partners.org

and iliotibial band (ITB) releases for refractory trochanteric bursitis.[5,6] As treatment of these tears evolved, open techniques emerged, though complication rates as high as 19% in some series were reported.[7] To further improve outcomes there has been increasing interest in endoscopic gluteal tendon repair, which as of yet has reported very low complication rates with tremendous gains in functional recovery.[8–12]

The gluteus medius and minimus span from the ilium to the greater trochanter. Innervated by the superior gluteal nerve, they serve as the primary abductors of the hip and are pivotal in stabilizing the pelvis during gait.[2,13] While in the stance phase of gait, the gluteal muscles are responsible elevating the contralateral hemipelvis as deficiency may lead to a Trendelenburg gait.[14] Therefore, repair of these muscles when ruptured can have a significant impact on a patient's ability to ambulate, and overall quality of life.

When considering surgical repair of the abductor tendons, an understanding of the anatomic attachments is essential as restoring the native anatomy is necessary to optimize function. These attachments are relatively complex as the gluteus medius and minimus each have multiple distinct insertion sites on the greater trochanter.[1,2,4,13] These may be better appreciated by awareness of the four facets of the greater trochanter: superoposterior, lateral, anterior, and posterior. The gluteus medius has one attachment to the superoposterior facet and another to the lateral facet.[1,2,4,13] Composed of three fiber groupings, the anterior and middle fibers attach to the lateral facet while the posterior fibers attach to the superoposterior facet.[2,13] The gluteus minimus also has two attachments as it traverses deep to the gluteus medius, inserting on the lateral facet and directly to the joint capsule.[1,2,4,13] It is important to note that there is a naturally occurring "bald spot" on the greater trochanter between the gluteus medius and minimus attachments.[2,13] Recognition of these landmarks with repair to the appropriate locations is crucial (**Fig. 1**).

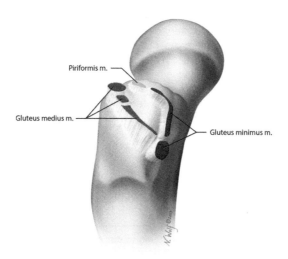

Fig. 1. Gluteal insertion sites on the greater trochanter. The anterior and central fibers of the gluteus medius attach to the lateral facet, whereas the posterior fibers attach to the superoposterior facet (*purple*). The gluteus minimus attaches on the anterior facet and joint capsule (*blue*). m, muscle. (*Courtesy of* Nicole Wolf, MS, Manchester, NH, with permission; nicolewolf@NicoleWolfArt.com.)

Gluteal tendon tears can occur acutely secondary to trauma or, more commonly, insidiously over time and may be misdiagnosed as trochanteric bursitis, hip arthritis, or lumbar disease.[1,2,4,13] Oftentimes they are elusive to clinical diagnosis with subtle gait alterations as hip abductor weakness occurs.[2,14] When hip abductor weakness progresses, significant alterations in gait may arise, including an abductor lurch; and an apparent leg length discrepancy may result from pelvic tilt. All of these factors greatly increase the forces placed on the spine and contralateral lower limb. MRI is diagnostic;[2,4] however, correlation with clinical findings is imperative as abductor tendon tears may be found incidentally in older patients[1] (**Figs. 2** and **3**). In cases involving symptomatic chronic tears, surgery is reserved for properly selected patients contingent on physiologic age, compliancy, and failure of conservative treatment[1,2,4,13,14] (**Box 1**). Patients with significant long-standing weakness and evidence of severe muscle atrophy/fatty infiltration by MRI are not considered surgical candidates.[2,14]

SURGICAL POSITIONING AND PORTAL PLACEMENT

The peritrochanteric space can be accessed from either the lateral decubitus or supine position. In the lateral decubitus, the patient is positioned with a bean bag or pegboard with the pelvis orthogonal to the floor. Slight abduction is applied to reduce tension on the ITB. The peritrochanteric space is first injected with an epinephrine-saline mixture to facilitate access into this potential space and improve hemostasis.[13] Direct lateral proximal and lateral distal portals are first established on either side of the trochanter as viewing portals. These portals should be created a few centimeters on either side of the trochanter, and approximate 45° angle to the insertion sites of the gluteal tendons on the greater trochanter.[1,13] The senior author prefers to use a 30° scope with a pump pressure of approximately 40 mm Hg.

The peritrochanteric space is further divided into superficial and deep regions. The superficial peritrochanteric space lies just beneath the subcutaneous tissue, but

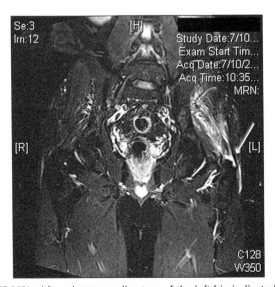

Fig. 2. Coronal T2 MRI with a gluteus medius tear of the left hip indicated by the white arrow. Detachment can usually be seen as the tendon retracts posterior and superior in this view. (*Courtesy of* Scott D. Martin, MD, Boston, MA.)

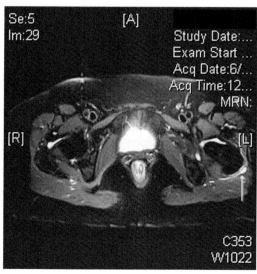

Fig. 3. Axial T2 MRI with a gluteus medius tear of the left hip indicated by the white arrow. Detachment can usually be seen as the tendon retracts posterior in this view. (*Courtesy of* Scott D. Martin, MD, Boston, MA.)

superficial to the musculotendinous sheath running down the lateral aspect of the thigh (**Fig. 4**, Video 1). This sheath is composed of the iliotibial band, tensor fascia lata, and gluteus maximus.[1,4] Advancement of the scope through this layer allows access to the deep peritrochanteric space which extends down to the greater trochanter (**Fig. 5**). Once in the deep peritrochanteric space, key structures should be identified including the gluteus medius and minimus tendons (proximal), gluteus maximus muscle belly and tendon (proximal and posterior), and the origin of the vastus lateralis (distal). Within this space also lies the trochanteric bursa, which may be secondarily inflamed.[1,3,4,13] Accessory portals can then be established as needed[7] (**Fig. 6**).

Gluteal Tendon Repair Technique

Gluteus medius and minimus repairs can be performed endoscopically in the deep peritrochanteric space. Patients are placed in the lateral decubitus position being sure to pad all bony prominences. The hip is placed in neutral rotation with neutral to slight abduction of the operative extremity. Initially the superficial peritrochanteric space is entered through two portals and the ITB is identified following which the deep peritrochanteric space is entered beneath the ITB. This technique can easily be done using fluoroscopic guidance to assist in portal placement with triangulation of the direct lateral proximal and distal portals directed at the gluteal tendon footprint with an ideal approach angle of 45° at the level of the skin to allow for enough working room. Accessory portals, such as the anterior portal, can then be established via direct visualization to aid in freeing up and reducing the torn tendon. The attachment sites for the gluteus medius and minimus tendons are isolated, and the torn tendon is identified observing that the tendon nearly always retracts posteriorly (**Fig. 7**). As a technical note, partial-thickness tears can be challenging from the onset as the remaining attached tendon limits the volume of the peritrochanteric space (**Fig. 8**). The footprint for the attachment sites is lightly debrided.[10,13]

Box 1
Presentation and management of abductor tendon tears

History

- Lateral hip pain and/or weakness
  - Exacerbated by activity or pressure
  - Gait alteration

- Often insidious onset

- Increasing prevalence by middle age

- Higher prevalence in women

Physical examination

- Pain to palpation over greater trochanter

- Decreased hip abduction strength

- Trendelenburg gait - contralateral pelvic drop through stance phase

- Abductor lurch - compensatory lean towards affected side to prevent pelvic drop

- Trendelenburg sign - inability to balance on affected leg with contralateral pelvic drop

Imaging

- Radiographs often unremarkable
  - Dystrophic calcification
  - Cortical changes at insertion

- Ultrasound can identify tears and secondary inflammation

- MRI is diagnostic (91% accurate, 73% sensitive, and 95% specific)
  - Full- and partial-thickness tears, degree of tendon retraction, and fat atrophy
  - Secondary bursitis

Management

- Trial of conservative management including physical therapy, NSAIDs, activity modification, and cautious anesthetic/corticosteroid injections

- Surgery if failed conservative management

Data from Refs.[1,2,4,13,14]

No two tendon tears are alike, and repair configuration should be developed based on that which will accurately restore the native anatomy. The authors prefer using a 5.5-mm triple-loaded suture anchor (**Fig. 9**). In this case the sutures are shuttled through the tendon and tied securely (**Figs. 10–15**, Videos 2 and 3).

For large full-thickness tears or in patients with a poor-quality tendon, a transosseous equivalent technique can be used for a more robust repair. If a transosseous equivalent technique is used, the senior author prefers a 5.5-mm triple-loaded suture anchor device for the proximal row. The tails of the sutures are then passed through the tendons and placed through push lock anchors (4.75 mm), which are inserted into the bone of the vastus ridge for a more secure repair (**Figs. 16–18**, Video 4). Patients are encouraged to use an abduction brace for one month and crutches with foot-flat progressive weight bearing as tolerated for six weeks. Progressive return to activity is allowed after three months when strengthening commences. Recent studies reviewing functional outcomes after endoscopic repairs have demonstrated excellent results[2,8–12] (**Table 1**).

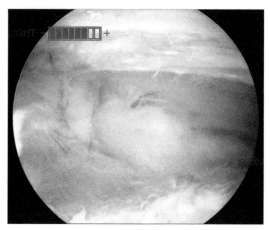

Fig. 4. ITB as seen from the superficial peritrochanteric space. (*Courtesy of* Scott D. Martin, MD, Boston, MA.)

COXA SALTANS

Coxa saltans (snapping hip syndrome) refers to snapping in or around the hip that can be due to multiple etiologies. The first key distinction is if the origin is intra- or extra-articular in nature. Intra-articular causes, such a labral tears, typically result in mechanical locking or catching within the joint with patients localizing pain to the groin. While important to consider, they are out of the scope of this article, as focus will be on extra-articular coxa saltans. It is important to note that intra- and extra-articular coxa saltans can occur simultaneously so thorough evaluation is crucial.[15–17]

Extra-articular coxa saltans is comprised of two distinct entities: coxa saltans interna and coxa saltans externa. Coxa saltans interna is attributed to snapping of the iliopsoas tendon, while coxa saltans externa is due to snapping of the posterior

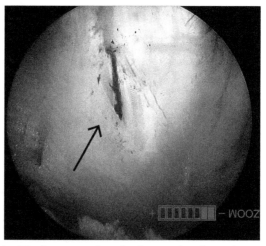

Fig. 5. Incision of the ITB allows entry into the deep peritrochanteric space. The black arrow is pointing to the incision in the ITB. (*Courtesy of* Scott D. Martin, MD, Boston, MA.)

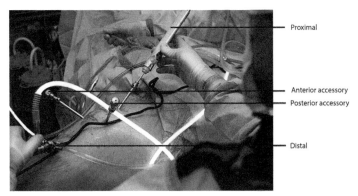

Fig. 6. Portal placement. Four portals are established in relation to the greater trochanter: direct lateral proximal and distal portals as well as anterior and posterior accessory portals. (*Courtesy of* Nicole Wolf, MS, Manchester, NH, with permission; nicolewolf@NicoleWolfArt.com.)

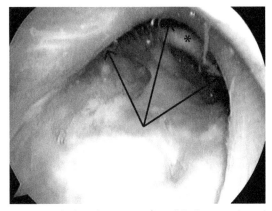

Fig. 7. Full thickness tears of the gluteus medius (*black arrows*) and minimus tendons (*asterisk*). For full-thickness tendon tear repair technique, see Video 2. (*Courtesy of* Scott D. Martin, MD, Boston, MA.)

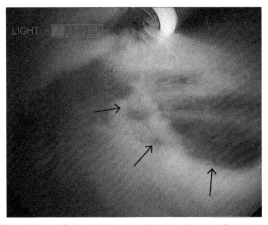

Fig. 8. Partial-thickness tear of the gluteus medius tendon as demarcated by the arrows. (*Courtesy of* Scott D. Martin, MD, Boston, MA.)

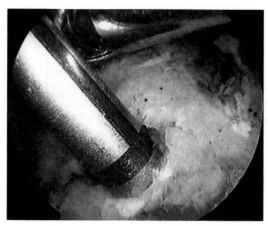

Fig. 9. Suture anchor placement in the gluteal tendon footprint. The anchor is inserted at a deadman's angle to prevent pullout of anchor. (*Courtesy of* Scott D. Martin, MD, Boston, MA.)

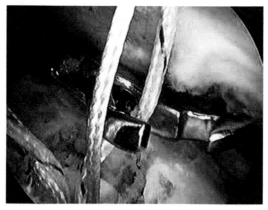

Fig. 10. A clever hook can be used to pass the suture through the gluteus minimus tendon. (*Courtesy of* Scott D. Martin, MD, Boston, MA.)

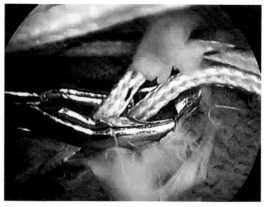

Fig. 11. After the minimus is repaired, an anchor is placed at the footprint of the gluteus medius and the suture is passed again with a clever hook. (*Courtesy of* Scott D. Martin, MD, Boston, MA.)

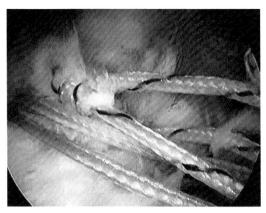

Fig. 12. Knots are securely tied. (*Courtesy of* Scott D. Martin, MD, Boston, MA.)

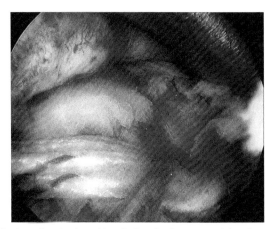

Fig. 13. A swivel lock anchor is placed just below in the vastus ridge for transosseous equivalent repair. (*Courtesy of* Scott D. Martin, MD, Boston, MA.)

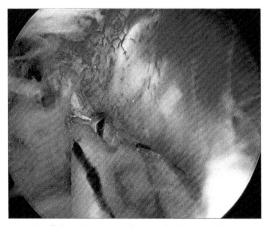

Fig. 14. Completed repair of the gluteus medius and minimus. (*Courtesy of* Scott D. Martin, MD, Boston, MA.)

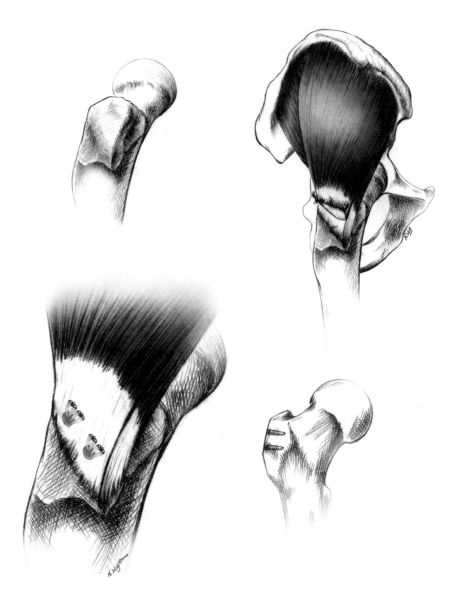

Fig. 15. Muscle attachments and completed single row repair. (*Courtesy of* Nicole Wolf, MS, Manchester, NH, with permission; nicolewolf@NicoleWolfArt.com.)

iliotibial band or anterior gluteus medius. Key to differentiating these etiologies is the location of symptoms, as coxa saltans externa presents with lateral snapping while coxa saltans interna occurs in the anterior groin. The presence of visual or auditory snapping can assist in making this distinction.[15,16] Symptomatic extra-articular coxa saltans is thought to more commonly occur in athletes, particular those participating in activities where the extremes of motion are frequently tested.[4,16] Though often benign, symptoms can be concerning to patients. Pain is often due to inflammation of the surrounding tissues, with most responding well to conservative treatment

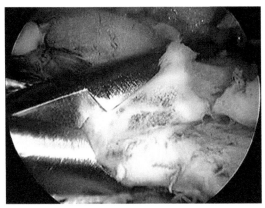

Fig. 16. A suture shuttle can be used to pass the suture through the gluteus medius tendon. (*Courtesy of* Scott D. Martin, MD, Boston, MA.)

including activity modification.[4,15,16] Coxa saltans interna and externa will each be discussed further.

Internal Coxa Saltans

Coxa saltans interna is characterized as snapping of the iliopsoas in the anterior aspect of the hip. Multiple etiologies have been proposed for the location of snapping, but it is thought to most commonly occur over the iliopectineal eminence (**Fig. 19**) or femoral head.[15,16] It may also occur after total hip arthroplasty if components are prominent or protrude out from beneath the anterior wall.[15] In contrast to coxa saltans externa, coxa saltans interna is less seldom visible though often audible.[15] Symptoms may be recreated by moving the patient's hip from flexion, abduction, and external rotation to extension, adduction, and internal rotation. Occasionally, simple hip flexion to extension with the patient supine can cause snapping. However, snapping can occur in any plane. Imaging rarely reveals abnormalities besides local inflammation. Ultrasound may identify abnormal movement of tissue.[15,10] Further exam findings can be found in **Box 2**. Though coxa saltans interna can be found in asymptomatic patients, treatment is only recommended if it is a source of pain.[15] If patients fail

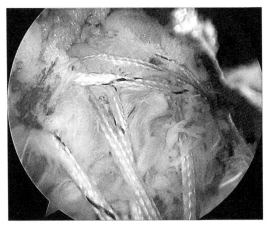

Fig. 17. Completed transosseous equivalent repair of the gluteus medius. (*Courtesy of* Scott D. Martin, MD, Boston, MA.)

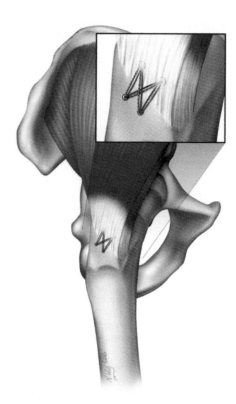

Fig. 18. The final transosseous equivalent repair. This method is often used for larger tears or patients with poor tendon quality. (*Courtesy of* Nicole Wolf, MS, Manchester, NH, with permission; nicolewolf@NicoleWolfArt.com.)

conservative treatment, including a stretching program, physical therapy, and steroid injections, they may be considered for iliopsoas tendon recession.[15,16] Iliopsoas dysfunction may be encountered with other concomitant hip disorders, such as femoroacetabular impingement or labral tears,[15,17] and result from caused by an antalgic or hip flexion gait. Patients may respond to conservative treatment once the inciting painful cause of hip discomfort is alleviated (**Box 2**).

Iliopsoas Tendon Recession

Iliopsoas tendon recession is not done routinely if there are no obvious signs of structural abnormalities of the tendon. However, it may be required for cases of recalcitrant snapping hip syndrome when other factors for hip pain have been ruled out. In cases of recalcitrant snapping hip syndrome, arthroscopic release of the iliopsoas tendon can be performed from an intra-articular position just medial to the anterior portal, in the peripheral compartment between the zona orbicularis and the labrum at the level of the medial synovial fold or endoscopically at the level of the lesser trochanter. Intra-articular releases are done by meticulously removing the overlying capsule and then recessing the tendon with electrocautery (**Fig. 20**, Video 5). Extra-articular release at the level of the lesser trochanter is done with two portals: one placed at the level of the lesser trochanter anterior to the femur and the second just distal to the lesser trochanter for use as the utility portal. Release is done with radio or electrothermal devices after

Table 1
Outcomes and complications reported with endoscopic abductor tendon repair

Study, Year	Level of Evidence	Mean Age (y)	Operative Hips	Mean Follow-up (mo)	Functional Outcomes (Preop to Postop)	Complications
Voos et al,[8] 2009	IV	50.4	10	25.0	All 10 patients regained 5/5 strength postop mHHS: 94 postop; HOS: 93	NR
Domb et al,[9] 2013	IV	58.0	15	27.9	RMC: 4.2–4.73; mHHS: 48.9–84.6; HOS-ADL: 47.47–88.1; HOS-SSS: 28.18–78.83; NAHS: 46.02–76.74	NR
McCormick et al,[10] 2013	IV	65.9	10	22.6	HHS: 84.7; HOS-ADL: 89.1; HOS-SSS: 86.8	NR
Thaunat et al,[11] 2013	IV	68.5	4	6.0	HHS: 35.7–74.0; NAHS: 38.3–83	NR
Chandrasekaran et al,[12] 2015	IV	57.0	34	24.0	Statistically significant improvement in mHHS, NAHS, HOS-ADL, HOS-SS	No repair failures; 4 hips went onto total hip arthroplasty (11–16 mo postop)

Abbreviations: HOS, hip outcomes score; HOS-ADL, hip outcomes score–activities of daily living; HOS-SSS, hip outcome score–sport-specific subscale; mHHS, modified Harris hip score; NAHS, non-arthritic hip score; NR, none reported; Preop, preoperative; Postop, postoperative; RMC, resisted muscular contraction score.
Data from Refs.[8–12]

isolating the tendon and maintaining meticulous hemostasis. A partial release is performed with the goal of lengthening the musculotendinous complex without losing the competency of the musculotendinous unit as would occur with complete release.

External Coxa Saltans

Coxa saltans externa is attributed to movement of the iliotibial band or gluteus maximus over the greater trochanter. Rarely traumatic, coxa saltans externa is frequently seen as an overuse injury with certain activities.[4,16] Diagnosis is often made by visualization of snapping over the lateral aspect of the hip as patients are able to recreate symptoms at will.[1] If not clearly visualized, palpating the greater trochanter while the patient flexes and extends may identify abnormal motion of tissue over the trochanter.[4] During hip flexion, the ITB lies anterior to the greater trochanter, moving posterior during extension.[4,15,16] Patients may describe a feeling as if their hip is "dislocating." Pain is due to inflammation of the local tissues, and a secondary bursitis may develop. Imaging is seldom abnormal except for signs of local inflammation.

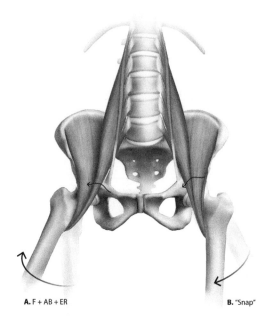

A. F + AB + ER   **B.** "Snap"

Fig. 19. Snapping of the iliopsoas tendon over the iliopectineal eminence can often be reproduced with patients lying supine as the leg is brought from flexion (F), abduction (AB), and external rotation (ER) to extension, adduction, and internal rotation. Arrows indicate direction of motion of various structures to evoke the snapping sensation of coxa saltans interna. (*Courtesy of* Nicole Wolf, MS, Manchester, NH, with permission; nicolewolf@NicoleWolfArt.com.)

Ultrasound may be used to identify catching of the tissues as they transverse the greater trochanter.[4,15,16] Further clinical evaluation and workup can be found in **Box 3**.

It is important to note that coxa saltans externa can occur in patients without pain. In these patients, no treatment should be pursued as it can be a normal finding. Treatment is only recommended when a source of pain, and most respond well to conservative management including rest, NSAIDs, stretching, steroid injections, and modification of activity upon return. Operative management entails ITB lengthening to reduce tension, but is reserved for refractory cases.[1,4,15,16] ITB lengthening will be discussed after ITB syndrome is addressed.

Trochanteric Bursitis

Isolated trochanteric bursitis is not common but is oftentimes associated with other disorders, such as gluteal tendon tears, lumbosacral disease, osteoarthritis of the hip, and overuse injuries, all of which may lead to an altered gait and development of trochanteric bursitis. Underlying conditions should always be addressed initially before any consideration for surgery.[4]

After diagnosis, patients should be treated conservatively with a minimum of two injections and a comprehensive physical therapy program targeting the core and hip musculature as well as a home stretching program. An MRI should be obtained; if there are loculations, thickened trochanteric bursa with edema, and evidence of ITB friction, surgical release may be considered after exhausting conservative treatment[4] (**Box 4**).

Box 2
Presentation and management of internal coxa saltans

History

- Snapping or catching sensation over anterior aspect of hip
  - Often audible

- Overuse injury

- Can occur after total hip arthroplasty if components protrude

Physical

- Symptoms recreated going from flexion to extension when supine

- Symptoms recreated with movement from flexion, abduction, external rotation to extension, adduction and internal rotation

Imaging

- Radiographs often unremarkable
  - Bony prominences, such as a cam lesion, may be identified

- Dynamic ultrasound may reveal snapping of tendon
  - Nonspecific signs of inflammation, tendon thickening, or secondary bursitis

- MRI often unremarkable, but can rule out other etiologies
  - Nonspecific signs of inflammation or secondary bursitis

Management

- Can be a benign finding, treat only if painful

- Often responds to conservative management
  - Stretching, activity modification, nonsteroidal antiinflammatory drugs, anesthetic/corticosteroid injections

- Surgical release/lengthening of iliopsoas tendon only if failed conservative management

Data from Yen YM, Lewis CL, Kim YJ. Understanding and treating the snapping hip. Sports Med Arthrosc 2015;23(4):194–9; and Lewis CL. Extra-articular snapping hip: a literature review. Sports Health 2010;2(3):186–90.

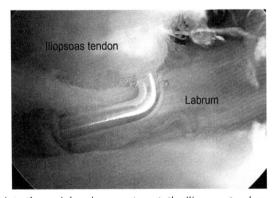

Fig. 20. On entry into the peripheral compartment, the iliopsoas tendon was found exposed and torn. Fraying of the underlying labrum from iliopsoas compression was also observed. The electrocautery probe is in the anterior portal, releasing the tendon as it enters the peripheral compartment over the labrum. (*Courtesy of* Scott D. Martin, MD, Boston, MA.)

Box 3
Presentation and management of external coxa saltans

History

- Snapping over lateral aspect of hip
  - May describe as *dislocating*
  - Frequently visible
- Overuse injury in active patients

Physical

- Patients often able to recreate with flexion/extension or abduction
- Snapping tissue palpated over greater trochanter as patient flexes and extends while in lateral decubitus position

Imaging

- Radiographs unremarkable
- Dynamic ultrasound can identify snapping tissue over the greater trochanter
  - Nonspecific signs of inflammation, tendon thickening, or secondary bursitis
- MRI often unremarkable
  - May reveal tendon thickening

Management

- Can be a benign finding, treat only if painful
- Frequently responds to conservative management
  - Physical therapy, stretching, activity modification, nonsteroidal antiinflammatory drugs, anesthetic/corticosteroid injections
- Surgical lengthening of ITB only if failed conservative management

Data from Yen YM, Lewis CL, Kim YJ. Understanding and treating the snapping hip. Sports Med Arthrosc 2015;23(4):194–9; Lewis CL. Extra-articular snapping hip: a literature review. Sports Health 2010;2(3):186–90; Strauss EJ, Nho SJ, Kelly BT. Greater trochanteric pain syndrome. Sports Med Arthrosc 2010;18(2):113–9; and Byrd JW. Disorders of the peritrochanteric and deep gluteal space: new frontiers for arthroscopy. Sports Med Arthrosc 2015;23(4):221–31.

Box 4
Presentation and management of trochanteric bursitis

History

- Insidious onset of lateral hip pain associated with overuse

Physical examination

- Pain on palpation over greater trochanter
- ITB tightness with Ober's test

Imaging

- Radiograph unremarkable
- Ultrasound may reveal inflammation of the ITB with secondary bursitis
- MRI unremarkable, but useful in ruling out alternate etiologies
  - Secondary bursitis

Management

- Nonoperative management
  - Stretching, activity modification, nonsteroidal antiinflammatory drugs, corticosteroid injections
- Surgery if symptoms fail to improve and no alternate source of symptoms identified

From Strauss EJ, Nho SJ, Kelly BT. Greater trochanteric pain syndrome. Sports Med Arthrosc 2010;18(2):113–9.

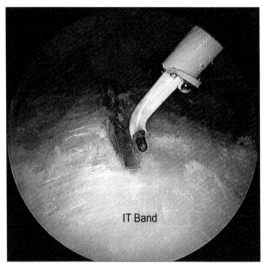

Fig. 21. Hook probe electrocautery is used for H-plasty of the ITB. Viewing from the distal portal with the electrocautery in the posterior portal, a longitudinal split is first made in the ITB. (*Courtesy of* Scott D. Martin, MD, Boston, MA.)

Iliotibial Band Release

ITB release is done endoscopically as a day surgery. The release can be done using 2 portals including the direct distal and proximal lateral portals. After obtaining visualization within the superficial peritrochanteric compartment, the ITB is recessed using an H-plasty technique,[1] which allows the ITB to expand around the greater trochanter without sacrificing the stability it provides during the gait cycle, and preserving the gluteus maximus attachment. A hook probe electrocautery device can be used to

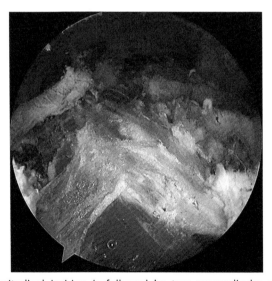

Fig. 22. The longitudinal incision is followed by two perpendicular cuts to complete the H-plasty being careful not to transect the ITB. (*Courtesy of* Scott D. Martin, MD, Boston, MA.)

		Mean		Mean		
Study, Year	Level of Evidence	Age (y)	Operative Hips	Follow-up (mo)	Functional Outcomes (Preop to Postop)	Complications
Ilizaliturri et al,[18] 2006	IV	26.0	11 Z-plasty	24.0	WOMAC: 81–94; all returned to full activity without pain; one had continued snapping	None
Farr et al,[19] 2007	IV	43.5	2 Released	41.0	All returned to full activity without pain	None
Govaert et al,[20] 2012	IV	NR	5 Released	1.5	VAS: 75–13 out of 100; WOMAC significantly improved	1 Hematoma requiring evacuation
Zini et al,[21] 2013	IV	25.0	15 Released	33.8	VAS: 5.5–0.53 out of 10; postop mHHS: 97.5; TAS: 7.6–7.6; 60% were pain free; all patients experienced relief of snapping; patient satisfaction: 9.3 out of 10	None

Abbreviations: mHHS, modified Harris hip score; NR, none reported; Preop, preoperative; Postop, postoperative; TAS, Tegner activity level scale; VAS, visual analog scale for pain; WOMAC, Western Ontario and McMaster Universities Osteoarthritis Index.
Data from Refs.[18–21]

efficiently perform the H-plasty in a precise fashion (**Figs. 21** and **22**, Video 6). Blood loss is minimal.

Patients are allowed immediate weight bearing with a cane or crutches for several days. Patients are taught a home stretching program with gradual return to all activities over three to four weeks. Full return to activity without pain is commonly reported (**Table 2**).

SUPPLEMENTARY DATA

Supplementary data related to this article can be found at http://dx.doi.org/10.1016/j.csm.2016.03.001.

REFERENCES

1. Byrd JW. Disorders of the peritrochanteric and deep gluteal space: new frontiers for arthroscopy. Sports Med Arthrosc 2015;23(4):221–31.
2. Lachiewicz PF. Abductor tendon tears of the hip: evaluation and management. J Am Acad Orthop Surg 2011;19(7):385–91.
3. Voos JE, Rudzki JR, Shindle MK, et al. Arthroscopic anatomy and surgical techniques for peritrochanteric space disorders in the hip. Arthroscopy 2007;23(11): 1246.e1241–5.

4. Strauss EJ, Nho SJ, Kelly BT. Greater trochanteric pain syndrome. Sports Med Arthrosc 2010;18(2):113–9.

5. Bunker TD, Esler CN, Leach WJ. Rotator-cuff tear of the hip. J Bone Joint Surg Br 1997;79(4):618–20.

6. Kagan A. Rotator cuff tears of the hip. Clin Orthop Relat Res 1999;368:135–40.

7. Walsh MJ, Walton JR, Walsh NA. Surgical repair of the gluteal tendons: a report of 72 cases. J Arthroplasty 2011;26(8):1514–9.

8. Voos JE, Shindle MK, Pruett A, et al. Endoscopic repair of gluteus medius tendon tears of the hip. Am J Sports Med 2009;37(4):743–7.

9. Domb BG, Botser I, Giordano BD. Outcomes of endoscopic gluteus medius repair with minimum 2-year follow-up. Am J Sports Med 2013;41(5):988–97.

10. McCormick F, Alpaugh K, Nwachukwu BU, et al. Endoscopic repair of full-thickness abductor tendon tears: surgical technique and outcome at minimum of 1-year follow-up. Arthroscopy 2013;29(12):1941–7.

11. Thaunat M, Chatellard R, Noel E, et al. Endoscopic repair of partial-thickness undersurface tears of the gluteus medius tendon. Orthop Traumatol Surg Res 2013; 99(7):853–7.

12. Chandrasekaran S, Gui C, Hutchinson MR, et al. Outcomes of endoscopic gluteus medius repair: study of thirty-four patients with minimum two-year follow-up. J Bone Joint Surg Am 2015;97(16):1340–7.

13. McCormick F, Martin SD. Endoscopic repair of the gluteus medius tendon. 2011. Available at: http://www.nicolewolfart.com/aaosGlutealRepair/martin_Gluteus MediusRepair.html. Accessed January 15, 2016.

14. Chandrasekaran S, Vemula SP, Gui C, et al. Clinical features that predict the need for operative intervention in gluteus medius tears. Orthop J Sports Med 2015; 3(2).

15. Yen YM, Lewis CL, Kim YJ. Understanding and treating the snapping hip. Sports Med Arthrosc 2015;23(4):194–9.

16. Lewis CL. Extra-articular snapping hip: a literature review. Sports Health 2010; 2(3):186–90.

17. El Bitar YF, Stake CE, Dunne KF, et al. Arthroscopic iliopsoas fractional lengthening for internal snapping of the hip: clinical outcomes with a minimum 2-year follow-up. Am J Sports Med 2014;42(7):1696–703.

18. Ilizaliturri VM Jr, Martinez-Escalante FA, Chaidez PA, et al. Endoscopic iliotibial band release for external snapping hip syndrome. Arthroscopy 2006;22(5):505–10.

19. Farr D, Selesnick H, Janecki C, et al. Arthroscopic bursectomy with concomitant iliotibial band release for the treatment of recalcitrant trochanteric bursitis. Arthroscopy 2007;23(8):905.e1–5.

20. Govaert LH, van Dijk CN, Zeegers AV, et al. Endoscopic bursectomy and iliotibial tract release as a treatment for refractory greater trochanteric pain syndrome: a new endoscopic approach with early results. Arthrosc Tech 2012;1(2):e161–164.

21. Zini R, Munegato D, De Benedetto M, et al. Endoscopic iliotibial band release in snapping hip. Hip Int 2013;23(2):225–32.

Ischiofemoral Impingement and Hamstring Syndrome as Causes of Posterior Hip Pain
Where Do We Go Next?

Hal David Martin, DO*, Anthony Khoury, MS,
Ricardo Schröder, PT, Ian James Palmer, PhD

KEYWORDS

- Ischiofemoral impingement • Hamstring syndrome • Posterior hip pain
- Deep gluteal syndrome • Sciatic nerve entrapment • Ischial tunnel • Hamstring tear

KEY POINTS

- Independently, or in combination, deep gluteal syndrome (DGS) can be associated with distal etiologies, such as hamstrings syndrome and ischiofemoral impingement.
- Six key physical examination tests are used to diagnose DGS, hamstrings syndrome, and ischiofemoral impingement when posterior hip pain is a complaint.
- Nonoperative and operative treatment planning is based on the differential diagnosis of posterior hip pain and the contributing pathoanatomy.

Recent advances in understanding the hip joint anatomy and biomechanics have contributed to the improvement of diagnosis and treatment decisions for deep gluteal syndrome (DGS).[1–5] Independently, or in combination, DGS can be associated with distal etiologies, such as hamstrings syndrome and ischiofemoral impingement (IFI). The presence of a scarred sciatic nerve (SN) to the hamstrings tendon, in cases of hamstrings syndrome, and SN impingement between the ischium and the lesser trochanter are isolated causes of posterior hip pain that can be distinguished between intrapelvic or extrapelvic SN entrapment.[3,6–10]

IFI and hamstrings syndrome are 2 sources of posterior hip pain that can simulate symptoms of DGS. These 2 dynamic pathologic conditions are associated with physical activity, and the coexistence of both conditions cannot be excluded.[3,10] To evaluate the etiology of posterior hip pain, it is necessary to understand, correlate,

Disclosure: The authors have nothing to disclose.
Hip Preservation Center, Baylor University Medical Center, 3900 Junius Street, Suite 705, Dallas, TX 75246, USA
* Corresponding author.
E-mail address: haldavidmartin@yahoo.com

and assess the interaction among the osseous, capsulolabral, musculotendinous, neurovascular, and kinematic levels. The combination of a comprehensive history and physical examination with imaging and ancillary testing are critical to diagnose DGS precisely.[3,5,10,11]

Johnson and Rochester[12] first described the surgical treatment for IFI in 1977, when noticing a narrowing ischiofemoral space associated with posterior hip pain after a total hip implant. The case was successfully treated with resection of the lesser trochanter. More recently, Hatem and colleagues,[4] in a 2-year outcome study, showed an improvement of the symptoms after partial lesser trochanterplasty in subjects diagnosed with IFI. Surgical procedures to treat chronic hamstrings tears and avulsions have reported positive outcomes in comparison with nonoperative treatment. Positive outcomes are also confirmed for surgical procedures to release scar tissue between the hamstrings tendons and SN.[2,8,13,14]

The goal of this article was demonstrate how to recognize and diagnose the distal causes of DGS. Readers will be able to distinguish independent IFI or hamstrings syndrome, which can exist with or without SN impingement.

ANATOMY AND BIOMECHANICS

The anatomic and biomechanical relationship of the SN to the proximal hamstrings insertion in the deep gluteal space is critical to diagnosis the distal causes of DGS. After exiting the pelvis anterior to the piriformis muscle, the SN runs posteriorly to the obturator/gemelli and quadratus femoris muscle, located at the most lateral aspect of the ischial tuberosity. The SN also maintains an intimate relationship with the hamstrings origin.[10,15] Within the ischiofemoral space, the SN shares the same spatial location with the lesser trochanter, which is separated from the SN by the quadratus femoris muscle.[10,15] The proximal insertion of the semimembranosus muscle at the lateral aspect of the ischium is another structure that shares the same anatomic spatial location within the ischiofemoral space. Distal to the ischium (7 cm from the ischial tuberosity), the first branch of the SN emerges adjacent to the long head of the biceps femoris, which can also contribute to SN entrapment as it courses to the lower extremity[9,15] (**Fig. 1**).

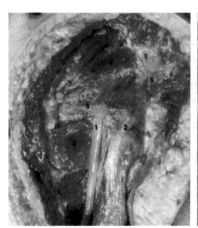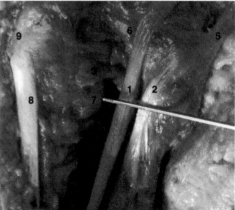

Fig. 1. Anatomy of the deep gluteal space. (1) SN; (2) conjoint tendon of semitendinosus and biceps femoris; (3) quadratus femoris muscle; (4) piriformis muscle; (5) sacrotuberous ligament; (6) obturator internus muscle; (7) lesser trochanter; (8) tensor fascia latae; (9) greater trochanter.

Located distally and medially to the sciatic notch, the sacrotuberous and sacrospinous ligaments have an important function in contributing to the symptoms of DGS and pudendal nerve entrapment.[16,17] The sacrotuberous ligament has extensions to the semitendinosus and biceps femoris tendon on the origin and share the same fascial insertion at the ischium. Tenderness or injuries of the sacrotuberous ligaments could be present in cases of chronic semitendinosus injuries and pudendal nerve entrapment.[18–20]

Isolated lesions in the proximal insertion of the hamstrings tendons can reproduce symptoms associated with DGS. Chronic and repetitive tears or a single acute lesion can contribute to the development of hamstrings syndrome.[9] In addition to the nature of the injury, traumatic or chronic, it is important to be aware of gluteal sitting pain.[3] Subjects with proximal hamstrings injuries may experience functional incapacity and pain at the ischium or lateral to the ischium with sitting, stretching, and during exercises, which is caused by SN traction, compression, or irritation.[9]

The development of extra-articular impingement with hip pain and kinematic compensation has been associated to abnormalities of the proximal hip morphology and its relationship with the ischiofemoral space.[3,21–23] In a study performed by Gómez-Hoyos and colleagues,[21,22] the femoral version and lesser trochanter version were compared between individuals with surgical confirmation of IFI versus asymptomatic subjects. Lesser trochanter angle does not show difference between groups; the symptomatic group showed significantly increased femoral anteversion and lesser trochanteric version angle (**Fig. 2**). Lesser trochanteric version alone does not influence the ischiofemoral space (IFS), the lesser trochanteric version may have an influence in subjects with chronic hamstrings tears, as observed clinically by the lead author (H.D. Martin). Further studies need to confirm these anatomic variations.

Tears in the proximal insertion of the hamstrings and lesser trochanteric impingement are 2 conditions that may coexist and simulate distal symptoms of DGS. Patti and colleagues[6] first reported these conditions in a case study of IFI. Posteriorly, Torriani and colleagues[7] showed that 5 of 10 subjects had a presence of proximal hamstrings tears associated with IFI. More recently, Gómez-Hoyos and colleagues[3]

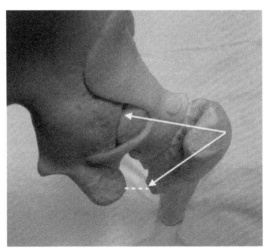

Fig. 2. Relationship of proximal femoral anatomy and the ischiofemoral space. (*Yellow arrows* represent the angle between the femoral version and lesser trochanteric version. *Dashed yellow* is the ischiofemoral space.)

used 17 subjects with IFI to validate the specificity and sensitivity of the long stride walking and IFI test to diagnose IFI. The population of the study showed as associated symptoms sitting pain (88.2%) and radiating pain (11.7%), 2 signs that have been consistently associated with DGS.

For the anatomy of the peritrochanteric space, the SN biomechanics should be understood. Normal hip joint motion results in a direct influence on neural tissue stretching, compression, and position. During straight leg raise, hip flexion with the knee in extension, the SN experiences an average of increased strain of 26%. The nerve also experiences proximal excursion the average of 28 mm at 70° to 80° of hip flexion.[24,25] As demonstrated in animal studies, the nerve conduction is completely blocked with 12% of strain, presenting minimal recovery after 1 hour.[26,27] Khoury and colleagues[28] showed that altering hip position in the frontal plane, increasing the hip abduction, decreased the strain parameters of the SN an average of 83.65%. In the same study, the investigators observed a "wrap-around" phenomenon, when the nerve spins on its axis during hip flexion. The investigators observed that the loss of the capacity to "wrap around" due to scars and entrapments may contribute to an abnormal nerve kinematics. The abnormal pathoanatomy not only affects the nerve impingement but can also affect the epineurial direction of normal nerve biomechanics. Restoring the normal SN excursion parameters are dependent on correcting the impinging pathoanatomy.

HISTORY AND PHYSICAL EXAMINATION

The assessment of posterior hip pain requires a complete history, comprehensive physical examination, and a standardized radiographic exploration to diagnose posterior hip pain precisely.[10,11] To evaluate the functional level of the patient and measure the outcomes of the treatment addressed, each patient undergoes a self-administered evaluation (International Hip Outcome Score and Harris Hip Score) as a part of the standard workup for posterior hip pain.[29]

Hamstrings syndrome and IFI can be associated with symptoms of DGS. Patients with SN entrapment often have a history of trauma and symptoms of sit pain (inability to sit for >30 minutes), radicular pain of the lower back or hip, and paresthesias of the affected leg.[9] As previously cited, patients with hamstrings syndrome and IFI can present radicular pain, and the coexistence of these conditions should be considered.[29]

The differential diagnosis of posterior hip pain can be localized to proximal or distal regions. Those producing distal SN impingement have different complaints from those who exhibit pain with walking or sitting. An example of pain exacerbated by sitting can include driving; when the hip is in 30° flexion, the hamstrings (semimembranosus) show a different force vector angle in comparison with 90° activation. Activities holding the hip in 30° hip flexion can reproduce SN complaints when the hamstrings are activated. Conversely, patients with IFI are more comfortable sitting, and walking during terminal hip extension when the space between ischium and the lesser trochanter is diminished, exacerbating the pain.[10,23] This diminished space is the location of the SN. If the normal biomechanics of this space is disrupted, the SN has the dynamic potential to be impinged.

The influence of limited hip range of motion on spine mobility and function has been shown as one of the causes of chronic low back pain.[30–34] Patients with IFI may present associated symptoms of low back pain due to the limited hip extension. This clinical observation was confirmed by Gómez-Hoyos[35] in a cadaveric study. Limiting hip extension by decreasing the ischiofemoral space resulted in increased intrafacet joint pressure of the lumbar spine (L3–L4 and L4–L5). A complete physical examination of the hip must comprise a lumbar spine evaluation; in the same way, cases of low back pain should also include a hip evaluation.

The physical examination to diagnose DGS, hamstrings syndrome, and IFI should be included in the standard hip joint evaluation protocol when posterior hip pain is a complaint (**Table 1**).[10,11] In the present work, a brief description of the key points and the main 6 tests previously validated to diagnose posterior hip pain are given. All hip joint evaluations should assess the 3 planar kinematic axes, comprising a gait analysis followed by an evaluation in the seated, supine, lateral, and prone positions.

The observation of the biomechanical axis alignment will provide information of the pelvic positioning. In normal osseous morphologic conditions, the balance between hip flexors and extensors influences the pelvic positioning in the sagittal axis. An abnormal pelvic positioning, posteriorly or anteriorly, has been associated with weakness and/or stiffness of the hip muscles involved with pelvic positioning, and this factor may contribute to the development of DGS and IFI.[36–39]

During the analysis of gait, the morphologic abnormalities of the hip joint, muscle weakness, pain patterns, and the long stride–walking test can provide important

Table 1
Steps for diagnosis and treatment of posterior hip pain

Condition	Diagnosis	Treatment
Ischiofemoral impingement	Assess structural contributing factors Distal pain lateral to the ischium Gait – Long stride walking (recreation of pain) vs short stride (alleviated pain) Ischiofemoral impingement test	• Nonoperative: ○ Abductor strengthening ○ Arch support ○ Injections ○ Limit stride length in sports and activities of daily living • Operative: ○ Open resection of the LT ○ Distalization of the LT ○ Ischioplasty: associated semimembranosus tear ○ Ischioplasty + LT resection: recreate normal ○ THA: associated osteoarthritis ○ Femoral osteotomy ○ Endoscopic LT resection
Hamstring syndrome	Pain lateral to the ischium Gait: heel strike (recreation of pain) Active hamstring test: 30° vs 90°	• Hamstring + IFI → ischioplasty + repair • Hamstring + sciatic nerve entrapment → open with neuromonitoring
Deep gluteal syndrome	Consider spine, SI, intrapelvis and gluteal space pathologies Pain proximal at the level of the piriformis Passive piriformis stretch test Active piriformis test	• Nonoperative: ○ Physical therapy: pelvic floor therapy ○ Guided injections ○ Steroids and neuromodulators • Operative: ○ Open sciatic nerve decompression ○ Intrapelvic laparoscopic decompression ○ Endoscopic decompression

Abbreviations: IFI, ischiofemoral impingement; LT, lesser trochanter; SI, sacroiliac joint; THA, total hip arthroplasty.

information to differentiate hamstrings syndrome and IFI. As previously cited, IFI was found to be more frequent in subjects with increased femoral version.[22,23] An internal foot progression angle during gait can present an increased femoral version and consequently is found with IFI.[22] A positive Trendelenburg sign can happen due to weakness of the gluteus medius muscle. A combination of hip adduction and pelvic tilt associated with rotational motion in axial load may contribute to lesser trochanteric impingement against the ischium, producing IFI symptoms.[10,22,23] The patterns of pain manifestation during gait can provide a key point for the diagnosis of posterior hip pain pathologies. During the initial heel strike, the hamstrings muscles act eccentrically, decelerating the leg during heel strike. Subjects referring pain lateral to the ischium during this specific motion may present a positive sign for proximal chronic or acute hamstrings tears. Differentially, the long stride–walking test is 1 of 2 tests used to diagnose IFI, and is a critical diagnosis tool.[3,4] Gómez-Hoyos and colleagues[3] showed this test with a sensitivity of 0.94 and specificity of 0.85 in the diagnosis of IFI. The long stride–walking test is positive when the patient refers pain lateral to the ischium during *terminal extension* that is relieved with short steps[4] (**Fig. 3**).

The palpation of the gluteal structures in the seated position using the ischial tuberosity as a reference point can also guide and distinguish sources of posterior hip pain[10] (**Fig. 4**). With the patient in sitting position, the active hamstrings test is performed. The patient is asked to actively flex the knee (positioned at 30° and 90° of

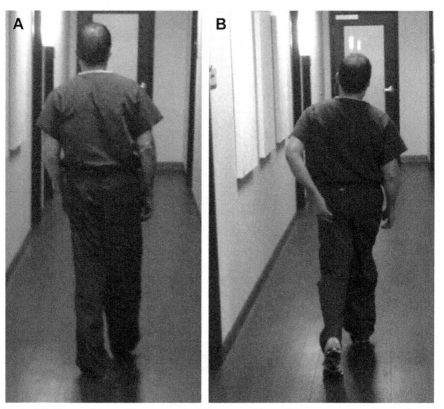

Fig. 3. (*A*) Short stride walking: no pain. (*B*) Long stride walking: recreation of pain lateral to the ischium.

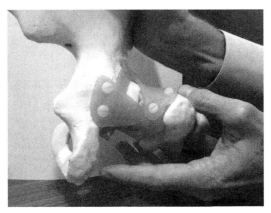

Fig. 4. Hand positioning for palpation of the deep gluteal space. From medial to lateral, the pudendal nerve entrapment is considered in cases of pain sensation medial to the ischium (1) in association with a tender sacrotuberous ligament, pain lateral to the ischium may represent hamstrings syndrome (2) or IFI (3), and finally, pain sensation at the sciatic notch characterizes the piriformis muscle (4).

flexion) against the resistance of the examiner. Reproduction of pain and/or complaint may represent a proximal hamstring tendon injury, hamstrings syndrome, and SN subluxation into the ischial tunnel.[10] Proximal from distal SN entrapment can be distinguished by the location of the symptomatic pain recreation.

From proximal to distal, the diagnosis of posterior hip pain can be differentiated through 2 tests in a seated position. The piriformis stretch test is performed (sensitivity of 0.52, specificity of 0.90) to diagnose DGS as the source of posterior hip pain. The test is performed with a flexion, adduction with internal rotation. The examiner extends the knee (engaging the SN) and passively moves the flexed hip into adduction with internal rotation while palpating the piriformis muscle lateral to the ischium or proximally at the sciatic notch. A positive test is the re-creation of the posterior pain at the level of the piriformis muscle lateral to the ischium or external rotators[5] (**Fig. 5**).

Finally, moving the patient to lateral decubitus, the last 2 tests to differentiate IFI and DGS are assessed. The active piriformis test showed sensitivity of 0.78 and specificity of 0.80 to diagnose DGS, and when used in association with the passive piriformis stretch test are major contributors to diagnose SN entrapment by the piriformis muscle. The patient is instructed to drive the heel into the examination table, initiating active hip abduction and external rotation against resistance from the examiner. Similar to the piriformis stretch test, a positive test is the presence of posterior pain at the level of the piriformis or external rotators.[5] While the patient is in lateral decubitus, the IFI test is performed. The pain is produced when the examiner extends the hip in association to adduction or in neutral position. To confirm the suspicion of IFI, the examiner extends the hip in neutral abduction with no symptom of pain, proving the presence of an impinging pathology. The IFI test showed a sensitivity of 0.82 and specificity of 0.85, and in combination with the long strides walking are used to identify IFI[3] (**Fig. 6**).

DIFFERENTIAL DIAGNOSIS

During the comprehensive history and physical examination, the examiner must be aware of DGS symptoms simulated by intrapelvic and extrapelvic structures. Cyclic

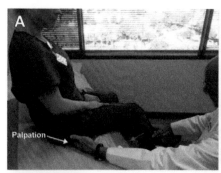

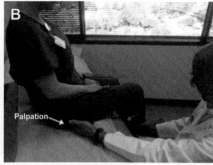

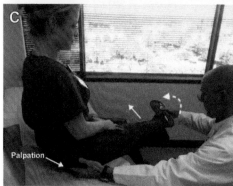

Fig. 5. Hamstrings active test and piriformis stretch test. (*A*) Active hamstrings test at 30° knee flexion. (*B*) Active hamstrings test at 90° knee flexion. (*C*) Piriformis stretch test. (*Red arrows*, active force by the patient against examiner resistance. *Yellow arrows*, the examiner places the hip into adduction and internal rotation.)

pain with a history of urogynecologic conditions (endometriosis, bladder or bowel issues, and dysmenorrhea) may indicate an intrapelvic SN entrapment.[10,16,17] Pudendal nerve entrapment is an isolated condition that may be associated with DGS that can be differentiated by a pain location and typical characteristics. Patients with pudendal nerve entrapment present with pain medial to the ischium and sensations of burning, tearing, stabbing lightninglike, electrical, sharp shooting, and/or foreign body sensation that is made worse with sitting (alleviated with toilet stool sitting) and reduced with standing.[17,40] The nerve can be entrapped in more than one location (piriformis, obturator internus muscles, sacrotuberous and sacrospinous ligaments, or the falsiform process), and a pelvic floor manual test performed by a trained physical therapist will assist the diagnosis and relationship of these intrapelvic conditions.[17,40,41]

IMAGING AND ANCILLARY TESTS

The standard imaging studies include the standing anterior-posterior pelvis, false profile, and lateral images. All intra-articular pathology is ruled out through a comprehensive history and physical examination assessing the 5 levels of osseous, capsulolabral, musculotendinous, neurovascular structures, and the kinematic chain. Specifically in posterior hip cases, the T3 MRI is performed to rule out intrapelvic sources of SN entrapment versus extrapelvic SN entrapment. The extrapelvic MRI patient positioning is important for IFI assessment. The feet are secured in a neutral walking position, which will most closely simulate a dynamic assessment of the ischiofemoral space. If the feet are not secured in this functional position, a false impression of

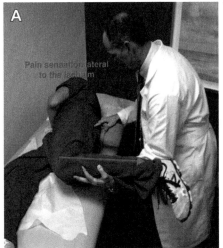
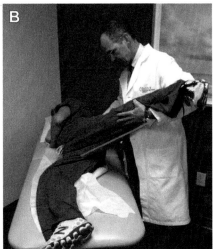
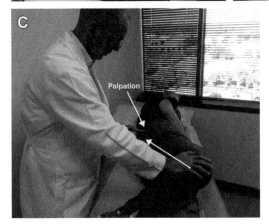

Fig. 6. Lateral position tests for differentiation of distal causes of DGS. Lateral position test. (*A*) IFI test the examiner moves the hip into extension (*red arrow*) in neutral or adduction (re-creation of pain lateral to the ischium); (*B*) The examiner moves the hip into extension (*red arrow*) with Abduction (alleviation of the symptoms abducting the leg); (*C*) Active piriformis test: the patient abducts and externally rotates the hip (*yellow arrow*) against the examiner resistance (*red arrow*) re-creation of pain lateral to the piriformis muscle helps to distinguish proximal from distal involvement etiologies.

decreased ischiofemoral space could occur. The assessment of the semimembranosus and its orientation to the lateral ischium is best visualized on T2 axial or T2 coronal imaging. This view allows for the detection of a partial tear or undersurface tears of the semimembranosus. In cases of active subluxation of the semimembranosus, dynamic MRI testing and dynamic ultrasound are useful. In dynamic ultrasound, the patient is placed in the prone position and the patient performs a bicycling motion with active hamstring contraction. The activated semimembranosus will sublux into the ischial tunnel recreating the radicular pain of the SN. Scarring in this region can be assessed by T1 and T2 MRI in the axial and coronal planes. The T3 MRI of the intrapelvis is used for gynecologic and vascular entrapments of the SN and/or its roots. This type of partial tear with subluxation into the ischial tunnel can be correlated with the physical examination assessment with the knee extended and the hip abducted.

Ancillary testing can include electromyography (EMG); however, it has not been found to be useful. If EMG is used, the testing should be performed in a dynamic modality with the knee in extension and the hip in flexion and abduction and the symptomatic side is compared with the nonsymptomatic side looking at neural latency.

Injection tests have been advocated for supporting the diagnosis of posterior extra-articular and intra-articular hip disorders. Anesthetic injection to the piriformis muscle can provide relief. Guided injections using computed tomography (CT), fluoroscopy, ultrasound, or MRI increase accuracy to the correct injection site. Ultrasound, as described previously, in addition to injection testing, is beneficial in the exact diagnosis of either IFI or hamstring tears involvement. Injection tests can include dynamic fluoroscopy to assess the IFS, or visualizing the dynamic recreation of the IF pain with the hip in terminal hip extension. Fluoroscopy can also be helpful in recreating greater trochanteric SN impingement, which can exist proximally. The ligamentous constraints of the hip do affect the overall kinematics of the hip and can affect the exact locations of impingement. This is evidenced through a multilayer effect, not just osseous but also capsulolabral, which can influence any of the other structures above or below the primary area of complaint.

TREATMENT
Nonoperative Treatment

The nonoperative treatment of posterior hip pain is a result of a comprehensive history and physical examination. A combination of physical therapy, nonsteroidal intramuscular injections, neuropsychological evaluation/treatment, and home exercises program are used as a standard protocol for nonoperative treatment.[10,41]

The physical therapy treatment for individuals with hamstrings syndrome, IFI, or DGS must involve associated factors such as lumbosacral spine alignment and stabilization, pelvic floor, and intra-articular structures. The intervention strategy for those with posterior hip pain is directed to rebalance the muscle-articular functioning of the hip/pelvis and spine through soft tissue mobilization, stretching and strengthening exercises, and aerobic conditioning. In cases of pelvic floor and urogynecological involvement, a pelvic floor therapy is applied to the treatment plan.

Nonsteroidal CT-guided injections are used as a diagnosis tool and treatment alternative. For those with DGS, IFI, and hamstrings syndrome, the utilization of injections can help to differentiate the source of pain, when correctly administered at the structure under investigation, producing relief of pain.[10,42,43] The posterior hip pain may have a chronic pathologic characteristic, affecting quality of life and mental health. A neuropsychiatric evaluation is required and a treatment is administered when appropriated.[41]

In addition to the clinical treatment, educational strategies addressing activities of daily living and a handout containing a home exercise program is delivered. The exercises are directed to increase the SN mobility into the deep gluteal space, combining the piriformis stretch, neural mobilization and SN–greater trochanter mobilization (hip circumduction) (**Fig. 7**).[41]

Surgical Treatment

In the event that a patient does not achieve pain relief with conservative treatment, surgical intervention is considered. The surgical treatment chosen will depend on both the clinical diagnosis and imaging evaluation, and to the patients' response to targeted injections during the conservative treatment stage.

The surgical treatment of DGS involving IFI or hamstrings avulsion must address the relevant pathology. The goal of surgery is to restore normal anatomy and normal neural function. The correct surgical procedure to address IFI encompasses the assessment of the entire biomechanical axis, as previously described. These procedures vary and include both open and endoscopic techniques to treat the conditions. Cases of IFI

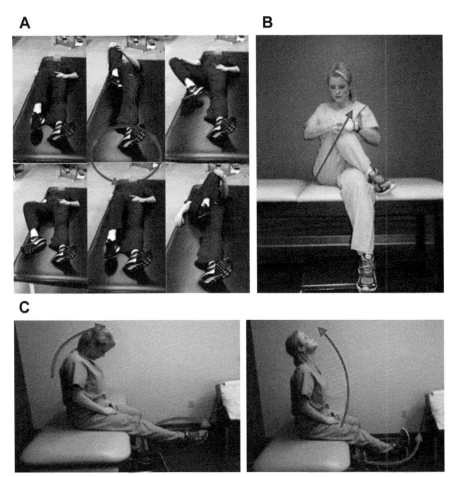

Fig. 7. Home exercise program. (*A*) Hip circumduction; (*B*) piriformis stretch; (*C*) neural mobilization. (*Red arrows*, direction of active motion by the patient.)

may be easily resolved with simple solutions, such as a shoe lift to moderate leg length inequality, or addressing a hyper-pronated hind foot by bringing the extremity into less internal rotation during midfoot stance phase. The presence of genu valgum or coxa valga may influence the IFS and result in painful pathologies. If the femoral torsion is greater than 30° of femoral anteversion, one must consider the need for a femoral de-rotational osteotomy, depending on the 3 planar osseous planar assessments. Each case should have a McKibbin index, acetabular and femoral version performed. The entire biomechanical axis in addition to the bimalleolar axis in determining the proper course of treatment is assessed. In cases of simple IFI that have failed conservative treatment, surgical intervention may be required.

The endoscopic technique was proven successful as reported by Hatem and colleagues[4] with the modified Harris Hip Score (mHHS), visual analog scale, and return to sport significantly improving after 2 years of follow-up. Surgical treatment for ischiofemoral impingement requires complete 3-planar valuation of the osseous anatomy involved with IFI. The endoscopic treatment options can involve open or endoscopic techniques to restore the normal anatomy. The goal is a functionally normal ischiofemoral space, the distance between the ischium and lesser trochanter. This may involve isolated lesser trochanterplasty and ischioplasty. The procedure is performed similar to Hatem and colleagues.[4] The patient is placed supine on a traction table with 20° contralateral tilt. Three portals are used: anterolateral, posterolateral, and auxiliary distal at level of lesser trochanter, as seen in **Fig. 8**. Traction is used for a maximum of 15 minutes while the intra-articular space was arthroscopically examined, with the remainder of the procedure performed without traction. A 70° high-definition arthroscope is used in the anterolateral portal, while the posterolateral and auxiliary distal portal are primarily used for a probe, arthroscopic burr, curved retractors, or arthroscope. Resection of the quadratus femoris is necessary to provide a window to access the lesser trochanter between the medial circumflex femoral artery and first perforating femoral artery. Lesser trochanteroplasty of the posterior one-third is then performed to obtain a functionally normal ischiofemoral space. Dynamic hip movements of adduction-extension and internal-external rotation are used to verify the lesser trochanter decompression.[4]

The cases presenting with hamstrings avulsions in conjunction with IFI can be addressed with a combination of ischioplasty and hamstrings repair, or with lesser trochanteroplasty. The goal is to recreate the standard IFS so as to achieve normal terminal hip extension, and to avoid any kinematic lumbar consequences. Identifying and decompressing the SN, which is often concomitantly involved, is critical to achieving optimal results. Chronic hamstring avulsions resulting in posterior hip pain can be repaired using an open or endoscopic approach. Full endoscopic approaches

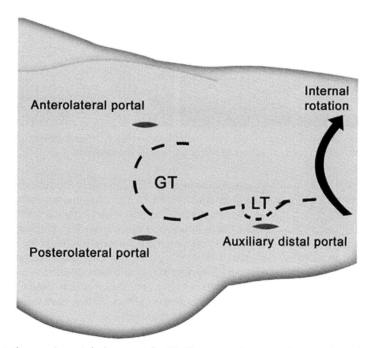

Fig. 8. Arthroscopic portal placement for IFI. Three portals are used: anterolateral, posterolateral, and auxiliary distal at the level of the lesser trochanter (LT). GT, greater trochanter. (*Reprinted from* Hatem MA, Palmer IJ, Martin HD. Diagnosis and 2-year outcomes of endoscopic treatment for ischiofemoral impingement. Arthroscopy 2015;31(2):241; with permission.)

to hamstring repair have increased in popularity due to complications associated with open techniques, including extensive tissue exposure, and proximity of incision to perianal zone[2,44]; however, the procedure becomes very difficult with retractions greater than 5 cm.[44]

The open approach for hamstrings avulsion is considered in late repairs, as there is a larger amount of scar tissue formation.[45] The patient is placed in the prone position with the knees in a flexed position. Depending on the amount of distal retraction, an incision may be either longitudinal or transverse to the gluteal fold. The fascia overlaying the hamstring compartment is exposed through blunt dissection of the subcutaneous tissue, and retraction of the gluteus maximus. Identification of the SN is necessary to prevent iatrogenic injury. The injured hamstrings tendons and anatomic insertion point of the common hamstrings tendon on the ischial tuberosity are identified. Following fibrous tissue debridement and suture anchor placement, the hamstrings are repaired. In the case of chronic tears, or tears older than 3 months, Achilles allograft tissue may be required.[45] The open surgical technique to treat hamstrings avulsions, both acute and chronic, is well documented, and it is recommended that a complete review of literature be performed to identify an appropriate procedure.[45–50]

An alternative approach is a mini-open surgical technique, which is assisted by dry endoscopy and neuromonitoring. The neuromonitoring reduces risk of intraoperative nerve damage.[51–53] The mini-open transgluteal approach is performed with the patient in a prone position. The ischial tuberosity and ischiofemoral space are identified under fluoroscopy, and an 8-cm transverse line is drawn. Hamstrings are accessed through the gluteus maximus two-thirds proximal and one-third distal to the muscle. The size and severity of hamstrings avulsion can then be monitored with the arthroscope through the incision. Once the degenerated tendon fibers and bursa are removed, the footprint of the torn tendon is decorticated with a 4.0-mm burr. Hamstrings reattachment to the normal anatomic footprint is performed with 4.5-mm sutures under direct fluoroscopic visualization.

The open technique may demonstrate a partially, but symptomatically, healed semimembranosus in partial healed and symptomatic avulsion. These avulsions are closed through the initial opening, which is easily identified in the partial tear once the small fibers are opened on the posterolateral corner of the ischium. The ischial angle also takes into consideration the degree of ischioplasty resection, with the overall goal of creating a flat surface by which the semimembranosus can be repaired with the recreation of the proper IFS. Should the ischium be resected, and the IFS is still diminished, it is recommended to internally rotate and approach the lesser trochanter through the central portion of the quadratus femoris.

Nerve mobility is assessed before closure and further adhesions, both proximally and distally, should be assessed. The wound is meticulously closed through the maximus fascia in addition to the subcutaneous tissue and a running subcuticular plastics closure. A sterile dressing is applied and left in place for the first 5 days. The knee is placed into flexion and remains in flexion throughout the closure. The knee is left in a locked position at 45° flexion for 3 to 4 weeks, or with more extension as tolerated by the SN. Physical therapy is initiated with the SN mobilization exercises as described in the following section.

Postoperative Treatment

The postoperative rehabilitation of IFI, DGS, and hamstrings syndrome surgeries represents a very important piece of treatment of posterior hip pain. The treatment

Table 2
Postoperative rehabilitation summary

Condition	Associated Findings	Specific Care	Time
IFI	• Limited hip extension; • Poor lumbopelvic stabilization; • Low back pain; • G. med + max. weakness; • Adductors contracture; • Increased femoral version.	• Neutral hip flexors stretching (0°) first 4 wk; • Crutches and partial weight bearing: 4 wk; • Lumbopelvic alignment and stabilization to control hip extension; • Immediate G. med + max. strengthening; • Reestablish the plantar arc (if necessary in cases of hyperpronation); • Avoid pelvic drop or lower extremity in excessive adduction and internal rotation during weight bearing.	12 (wk)
Hamstring syndrome	• Hamstring weakness associated with tendon retractions (in case of complete rupture); • Decreased SN mobility; • G. max weakness; • Altered pelvic sagittal alignment (anteriorly or posteriorly)	• Neutral hip flexors stretching (0°): 4 wk; • Lumbopelvic alignment and stabilization; • Crutches (6–8 wk) + flat foot during gait; • Knee brace locked between 30° and 45° flexion (45° during exercises): gradual extension with patient tolerance; • Sciatic nerve mobilization exercises in cases of scars between HS and SN; • First 3 wk: short stride walking; • Full ROM: 6 wk = hamstring strengthening.	24 wk–1 y
DGS	• Low back pain; • Piriformis and/or obturator internus contracture; • Pelvic floor issues; • External rotators weakness; • Femur in excessive adduction and internal rotation during functional activities;	• Neutral hip flexors stretching (0°): 4 wk; • Lumbopelvic alignment and stabilization; • Avoid neurapraxia: constant neural mobilization; • Crutches (6–8 wk) + flat foot during gait; • Knee brace locked between 30° and 45° flexion (45° during exercises): gradual extension with patient tolerance; • Passive distal (cervical and ankle) nerve glides: week 2, increase tension with patient pain tolerance; • After week 3, increase 10° knee extension per week (patient pain tolerance); • Total hip/knee ROM: week 8.	24 wk–2 y

Abbreviations: DGS, deep gluteal syndrome; G max, gluteus maximus; G med, gluteus maximus; HS, hamstring; IFI, ischiofemoral impingement; ROM, range of motion; SN, sciatic nerve.

strategy follows the same concept based on the preoperative findings and approaches.

The therapist should be comfortable with the anatomy and biomechanics of the repaired tissues, as previously was demonstrated the intimate relationship between those structures in the deep gluteal space. Strategies directed to improve the lumbo-pelvic stabilization, maintaining and increasing the SN mobility into the deep gluteal space are the overall goals for those conditions. **Table 2** summarizes the key points to follow in the postoperative rehabilitation.

SUMMARY

In conclusion, IFI and hamstrings avulsions involving the SN are recognized through a comprehensive history and physical examination using ancillary testing and 3 planar radiographic assessments. Outcomes are dependent on patient compliance and the understanding of the entire anatomy, biomechanics, clinical presentation, and open versus endoscopic treatment options.

REFERENCES

1. Martin HD, Shears SA, Johnson JC, et al. The endoscopic treatment of sciatic nerve entrapment/deep gluteal syndrome. Arthroscopy 2011;27(2):172–81.
2. Gómez-Hoyos J, Reddy M, Martin HD. Dry endoscopic-assisted mini-open approach with neuromonitoring for chronic hamstring avulsions and ischial tunnel syndrome. Arthrosc Tech 2015;4(3):e193–9.
3. Gomez-Hoyos J. Martin R. Schroder R. et al. Accuracy of two clinical tests for ischiofemoral impingement in patients with posterior hip pain and endoscopically confirmed diagnosis. Arthroscopy, in press.
4. Hatem MA, Palmer IJ, Martin HD. Diagnosis and 2-year outcomes of endoscopic treatment for ischiofemoral impingement. Arthroscopy 2015;31(2):239–46.
5. Martin HD, Kivlan BR, Palmer IJ, et al. Diagnostic accuracy of clinical tests for sciatic nerve entrapment in the gluteal region. Knee Surg Sports Traumatol Arthrosc 2014;22(4):882–8.
6. Patti JW, Ouellette H, Bredella MA, et al. Impingement of lesser trochanter on ischium as a potential cause for hip pain. Skeletal Radiol 2008;37(10):939–41.
7. Torriani M, Souto SCL, Thomas BJ, et al. Ischiofemoral impingement syndrome: an entity with hip pain and abnormalities of the quadratus femoris muscle. AJR Am J Roentgenol 2009;193(1):186–90.
8. Orava S. Hamstring syndrome. Oper Tech Sports Med 1997;5(3):143–9.
9. Young IJ, van Riet RP, Bell SN. Surgical release for proximal hamstring syndrome. Am J Sports Med 2008;36(12):2372–8.
10. Martin HD, Reddy M, Gomez-Hoyos J. Deep gluteal syndrome. J Hip Preserv Surg 2015;2(2):99–107.
11. Martin HD, Palmer IJ. History and physical examination of the hip: the basics. Curr Rev Musculoskelet Med 2013;6:219–25.
12. Johnson K, Rochester M. Impingement of the lesser after on the ischial ramus total. J Bone Joint Surg Am 1977;59(2):268–9.
13. Miller BSL, Gill J, Webb GR. The proximal origin of the hamstrings and surrounding anatomy encountered during repair. J Bone Joint Surg Am 2007;89-A(805):44–8.
14. Dierckman BD, Guanche CA. Endoscopic proximal hamstring repair and ischial bursectomy. Arthrosc Tech 2012;1(2):e201–7.

15. Miller SL, Webb GR. The proximal origin of the hamstrings and surrounding anatomy encountered during repair. Surgical technique. J Bone Joint Surg Am 2008; 90(Suppl 2):108–16.

16. Hibner M, Desai N, Robertson LJ, et al. Pudendal neuralgia. J Minim Invasive Gynecol 2010;17(2):148–53.

17. Filler AG. Diagnosis and treatment of pudendal nerve entrapment syndrome subtypes: imaging, injections, and minimal access surgery. Neurosurg Focus 2009; 26(2):E9.

18. Beltran L, Ghazikhanian V, Padron M, et al. The proximal hamstring muscle-tendon-bone unit: a review of the normal anatomy, biomechanics, and pathophysiology. Eur J Radiol 2012;81(12):3772–9.

19. Bierry G, Simeone FJ, Borg-Stein JP, et al. Sacrotuberous ligament: relationship to normal, torn, and retracted hamstring tendons on MR images. Radiology 2014;271(1):162–71.

20. Mercer SR, Woodlai SJ, Kennedi E. Anatomy in practice?: the sacrotuberous ligament. NZ J Physiother 2005;33(3):91–4.

21. Gomez-Hoyos J, Schroder R, Reddy M, et al. Is there a relationship between psoas impingement and increased trochanteric retroversion? J Hip Preserv Surg 2015;2(2):164–9.

22. Gómez-Hoyos J, Schroder R, Reddy M, et al. Femoral neck anteversion and lesser trochanter retroversion in patients with ischiofemoral impingement: a case-control magnetic resonance imaging study. Arthroscopy 2015. http://dx.doi.org/10.1016/j.neuron.2014.02.016.

23. Schroder R, Reddy M, Hatem M, et al. A MRI study of the lesser trochanteric version and its relationship to proximal femoral osseus anatomy. J Hip Preserv Surg 2015;1–7. http://dx.doi.org/10.1093/jhps/hnv067.

24. Coppieters MW, Alshami AM, Babri AS, et al. Strain and excursion of the sciatic, tibial, and plantar nerves during a modified straight leg raising test. J Orthop Res 2006;24:1883–9.

25. Coppieters MW, Andersen LS, Johansen R, et al. Excursion of the sciatic nerve during nerve mobilization exercises: an in vivo cross-sectional study using dynamic ultrasound imaging. J Orthop Sports Phys Ther 2015;45(10):731–7.

26. Wall EJ, Massie JB, Kwan MK, et al. Changes in nerve conduction under tension. J Bone Joint Surg Br 1992;74-B(1):126–9.

27. Boyd BS, Puttlitz C, Gan J, et al. Strain and excursion in the rat sciatic nerve during a modified straight leg raise are altered after traumatic nerve injury. J Orthop Res 2005;23(4):764–70.

28. Khoury A. Schroder R. Gomez-Hoyos J. et al. The effects of hip abduction on sciatic nerve biomechanics during terminal hip flexion. ISHA - Int Meet. Cambridge (United Kingdom): September 24–26, 2015.

29. Mohtadi NGH, Griffin DR, Pedersen ME, et al. The development and validation of a self-administered quality-of-life outcome measure for young, active patients with symptomatic hip disease: the international hip outcome tool (iHOT-33). Arthroscopy 2012;28(5):595–610.e1.

30. Ellison JB, Rose SJ, Sahrmann S. Patterns of hip rotation range of motion: a comparison between healthy subjects and patients with low back pain. Phys Ther 1990;70(9):537–41.

31. Cibulka MT, Sinacore DR, Cromer GS, et al. Unilateral hip rotation range of motion asymmetry in patients with sacroiliac joint regional pain. Spine J 1998;23(9):971–1082.

32. Vad VB. Low back pain in professional golfers: the role of associated hip and low back range-of-motion deficits. Am J Sports Med 2004;32(2):494–7.

33. Van Dillen LR, Gombatto SP, Collins DR, et al. Symmetry of timing of hip and lumbopelvic rotation motion in 2 different subgroups of people with low back pain. Arch Phys Med Rehabil 2007;88(3):351–60.

34. Van Dillen LR, Bloom NJ, Gombatto SP, et al. Hip rotation range of motion in people with and without low back pain who participate in rotation-related sports. Phys Ther Sport 2008;9(2):72–81.

35. Gómez-Hoyos J, Khoury A, Schroder R, et al. The hip-spine effect: A cadaveric study of ischiofemoral impingement in hip extension effecting loads in lumbar facet joints. Arthroscopy, in press.

36. Halbertsma JP, Göeken LN, Hof AL, et al. Extensibility and stiffness of the hamstrings in patients with nonspecific low back pain. Arch Phys Med Rehabil 2001;82(2):232–8.

37. Neumann DA. Kinesiology of the hip: a focus on muscular actions. J Orthop Sports Phys Ther 2010;40(2):82–94.

38. Ekstrom RA, Donatelli RA, Carp KC. Electromyographic analysis of core trunk, hip, and thigh muscles during 9 rehabilitation exercises. J Orthop Sports Phys Ther 2007;37(12):754–62.

39. Sullivan MK, Dejulia JJ, Worrell TW. Effect of pelvic position and stretching method on hamstring muscle flexibility. Med Sci Sports Exerc 1992;24(12):1383–9.

40. FitzGerald MP, Kotarinos R. Rehabilitation of the short pelvic floor. II: Treatment of the patient with the short pelvic floor. Int Urogynecol J Pelvic Floor Dysfunct 2003; 14(4):269–75 [discussion: 275].

41. Schroder R. Gomez-Hoyos J. Martin R. et al. Non-operative treatment of deep gluteal pain: a case series of seven patients. ISHA - Int Meet. Cambridge (United Kingdom): September 24–26, 2015.

42. Michel F, Decavel P, Toussirot E, et al. Piriformis muscle syndrome: diagnostic criteria and treatment of a monocentric series of 250 patients. Ann Phys Rehabil Med 2013;56(5):371–83.

43. Fishman LM, Dombi GW, Michaelsen C, et al. Piriformis syndrome: diagnosis, treatment, and outcome–a 10-year study. Arch Phys Med Rehabil 2002;83(3): 295–301.

44. Guanche CA. Hamstring injuries. J Hip Preserv Surg 2015;2(2):116–22.

45. Fetzer GB, Fischer DA. Hamstrings injuries. In: Guanche C, editor. Hip and pelvis injuries in sports medicine. 1st edition. Philadelphia: Lippincott Williams & Wilkins; 2010. p. 181–92.

46. Mica L, Schwaller A, Stoupis C, et al. Avulsion of the hamstring muscle group: a follow-up of 6 adult non-athletes with early operative treatment: a brief report. World J Surg 2009;33(8):1605–10.

47. Sallay P, Ballard G, Hamersly S, et al. The effect of collar on aseptic loosening and proximal femoral bone resorption in hybrid total hip arthroplasty. Orthopedics 2008;31(3):227.

48. Lempainen L, Sarimo J, Mattila K, et al. Proximal hamstring tendinopathy: results of surgical management and histopathologic findings. Am J Sports Med 2009; 37(4):727–34.

49. Chakravarthy J, Ramisetty N, Pimpalnerkar A, et al. Surgical repair of complete proximal hamstring tendon ruptures in water skiers and bull riders: a report of four cases and review of the literature. Br J Sports Med 2005;39(8):569–72.

50. Cross M, Vandersluis R, Wood D, et al. Surgical repair of chronic complete hamstring rupture in the adult patient. Am J Sports Med 1998;26(6):785–8.

51. Porat M, Orozco F, Goyal N, et al. Neurophysiologic monitoring can predict iatrogenic injury during acetabular and pelvic fracture fixation. HSS J 2013;9(3): 218–22.
52. Calder HB, Mast J, Johnstone C. Intraoperative evoked potential monitoring in acetabular surgery. Clin Orthop Relat Res 1994;305:160–7.
53. Baumgaertner MR, Wegner D, Booke J. SSEP monitoring during pelvic and acetabular fracture surgery. J Orthop Trauma 1994;8:127–33.

Avoiding Failure in Hip Arthroscopy

Complications, Pearls, and Pitfalls

Matthew Tyrrell Burrus, MD[a], James B. Cowan, MD[b],
Asheesh Bedi, MD[c],*

KEYWORDS

- Hip arthroscopy • Complication • Revision • Indication • Failure

KEY POINTS

- Neurapraxias are one of the most common complications following hip arthroscopy, but most are expected to resolve with time.
- Limiting traction time to 1 hour, with an absolute maximum of no greater than 2 hours, will likely reduce the incidence of neurapraxias and skin breakdown.
- Careful insertion of arthroscopic instruments will help to avoid traumatic injuries to intra-articular structures and chondral surfaces.
- Proper patient selection is key to optimizing the chance for a successful postoperative outcome.
- There is a substantial learning curve for hip arthroscopy and receiving specialized training likely helps to reduce the duration of this curve.

INTRODUCTION

Hip arthroscopy continues to gain popularity as a treatment option for a variety of hip pathologies. A recent national database study demonstrated a 250% increase in hip arthroscopic procedures between 2007 and 2011.[1] Likewise, the indications for hip arthroscopy continue to increase as surgeons become more comfortable with the technology and instrumentation and techniques continue to improve. However, the growth in case volume and innovation has been accompanied by a parallel rise in complications. Postoperative failures are likely multifactorial, with poor patient selection and incorrect diagnoses among the most common contributory factors. In

Disclosure Statement: The authors have nothing to disclose.
[a] Department of Orthopaedic Surgery, University of Virginia Health System, PO Box 801016, Charlottesville, VA 22911, USA; [b] Department of Orthopaedic Surgery, University of Michigan, 24 Frank Lloyd Wright Drive, Lobby A, PO Box 391, Ann Arbor, MI 48106, USA; [c] Sports Medicine, Orthopaedic Surgery, MedSport, University of Michigan, 24 Frank Lloyd Wright Drive, Lobby A, PO Box 391, Ann Arbor, MI 48106, USA
* Corresponding author.
E-mail address: ABEDI@med.umich.edu

Clin Sports Med 35 (2016) 487–501
http://dx.doi.org/10.1016/j.csm.2016.02.011
0278-5919/16/$ – see front matter © 2016 Elsevier Inc. All rights reserved.

this article, the various complications are discussed as well as tips to avoid them. Additionally, reasons for postoperative clinical failure are examined.

COMPLICATIONS

As with most orthopedic procedures, the complications from hip arthroscopy are diverse and difficult to accurately quantify. When all adverse events are included, an estimated 1.4% to 6.1% of patients will encounter at least 1 complication from hip arthroscopy.[2–5] Fortunately, most of these complications are transient and do not likely impact long-term outcomes.[2,6,7] Included in this list are nerve and vascular injuries and iatrogenic damage to chondrolabral structures, as well as the less commonly seen hip destabilization, loose foreign body formation, skin damage, heterotopic ossification, and abdominal compartment syndrome.

Nerve Dysfunction

Of all complications, nerve dysfunction is the most commonly discussed, with neurapraxias, nerve compression, and direct nerve injury all potential mechanisms.[2,4,6–8] The lateral femoral cutaneous nerve (LFCN) and femoral nerve are at greatest risk when portals are created anterior to the greater trochanter. The pudendal nerve may be compressed between the pubic rami and perineal post, and the sciatic nerve may be stretched while traction is applied or directly injured during the creation of portals posterior to the greater trochanter. Although the frequency of these complications is likely underreported, most studies place the incidence at 1% to 10%.[2,7] However, a retrospective study by Dippmann and colleagues[7] specifically examined postoperative nerve symptoms and found that 46% (23/50) of patients had nerve dysfunction, but only 18% (9/50) persisted longer than 1 year. Similarly, Pailhé and colleagues[6] noted complete resolution of all pudendal neuralgias between 6 weeks and 3 months postoperatively.

To minimize traction-related nerve complications, the following recommendations have been made[6,8]:

- Lateral decubitus positioning
- A large, well-padded perineal post (8–10 cm) positioned just lateral to the patient's midline toward the operative extremity, which allows the minimum amount of traction necessary
- Distraction via an external distractor
- Generous systemic muscle relaxation
- Less than 50 pounds of traction
- Traction time less than 1 hour, with an absolute limit of 2 hours has been suggested. (Traction time may be minimized by removing the force during prepping and draping and after completion of treatment of central compartment pathology.)

However, as has been seen in previous studies, Dippmann and colleagues[7] noted no significant difference in traction time between patients with and those nerve dysfunction postoperatively (98 vs 100 min, $P = .88$), suggesting that traction is likely only one component of the overall risk. Merrell and colleagues[8] described their positioning technique using a taped, deflated beanbag instead of a perineal post and had zero cases of nerve dysfunction after 30 arthroscopic procedures.

To avoid direct injuries to nerves, careful portal creation and a knowledge of the path of the nerves is imperative (**Fig. 1**). To minimize nerve lacerations, only the skin should be cut with the scalpel followed by blunt penetration of the underlying soft tissues with the trocar and obturator. In 1995, Byrd and colleagues[9] published their findings from a

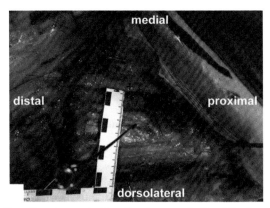

Fig. 1. Cadaveric dissection demonstrating the close proximity of the femoral neurovascular bundle to anterior hip arthroscopic portals (femoral nerve [+], femoral artery [*], and femoral vein [→]). (*From* Thorey F, Ezechieli M, Ettinger M, et al. Access to the hip joint from standard arthroscopic portals: a cadaveric study. Arthroscopy 2013;29(8):1297–307; with permission.)

cadaveric study examining the relationship between important neurovascular structures and commonly used arthroscopic portals. The LFCN is most susceptible to direct injury due to its location on the proximal thigh and because it has many branches that increase the chances of injury.[9–11] After the LFCN crosses under the inguinal ligament, it continues distally with variable arborization, as 1 in 4 nerves actually divide proximal to the inguinal ligament.[11] This places it, or one of its branches, within 3 mm of the anterior portal.[9] Use of a modified anterior portal that is slightly more lateral and distal can help to reduce this risk. Byrd and colleagues[9] noted that in their 8 cadaveric specimens, the LFCN had already divided into 3 or more branches at the level of the anterior portal. The femoral nerve was an average minimum distance of 3.2 cm from the anterior portal with the sciatic nerve 2.9 cm from the posterior portal. These numbers are slightly lower than what was found by Thorey and colleagues[12] in a similar study that also noted that the superior gluteal nerve was a mean distance of 20 ± 4 mm from the proximal anterolateral portal. To complicate this issue, Watson and colleagues[10] performed an MRI study on 100 patients to evaluate the course of the LFCN, femoral artery and nerve, and sciatic nerve in relation to various bony landmarks around the hip and noted that significant anatomic variations were seen in these structures when comparing patients of differing weights, body mass indices, and race.

Arterial Injury

Arterial injuries are much less common than nerve injuries, likely due to the larger margin of safety from the typical arthroscopic portals. The major blood vessels at risk are the femoral artery, ascending branch of the lateral femoral circumflex artery, and superior gluteal artery. At the level of the greater trochanter, the femoral artery lies 26 mm medial to a vertical reference line drawn from the anterior superior iliac spine.[10] The anterior peripheral portal is approximately 40 ± 16 mm from the lateral femoral circumflex artery, and the proximal anterolateral portal lies 20 ± 4 mm from the superior gluteal artery.[12]

Chondrolabral Damage

Because of the difficulty with accurately assessing bony landmarks and the depth of the joint compared with other joints, the hip cartilage and labrum are particularly at risk for injury during portal creation. They are especially vulnerable in hips with global or focal overcoverage and/or limited distraction despite traction. In their series of 250 patients, Badylak and Keene[13] noted a 20% (50/250) incidence of labral penetration by the localization needle, but they also demonstrated that these patients had no worse outcomes than those without labral penetration. However, Domb and colleagues[14] noted only a 0.67% (2/300) incidence of labral injury. Several techniques have been described to avoid this complication[4,14,15]:

- Apply traction before insertion of the needle.
- Once the needle penetrates the capsule, the intra-articular suction will be released, and then the femoral head distraction will increase.
- Initially, rotate the needle bevel toward the femoral head to minimize scuffing. Following joint venting, reinsert the needle with the bevel facing the labrum to avoid damaging the labrum. Once again, rotate the needle to have the bevel facing the head during insertion to protect the femoral cartilage.
- Use tactile feedback to guide cannula placement. It will slide easily through the capsule but not easily through the labrum.

Instrument Breakage

Instrument breakage resulting in loose foreign bodies is an uncommon complication of hip arthroscopy. Given the depth of the hip joint and the muscularity of the surrounding structures, accurate portal placement is crucial to avoid placing unnecessary torque on instruments. A review of 1054 consecutive hip arthroscopies included only 2 instances of instrument breakage.[2] In one case, a fragment broke off of the arthroscope within the joint, and the other case involved the metal jaw of a grasping forceps breaking during removal of a loose body. Another review of hip arthroscopy complications in children and adolescents found one instance of instrument breakage among 218 arthroscopies.[16] Although these studies did not discuss or evaluate the cause for instrument breakage, surgeons should always handle arthroscopic instruments delicately and inspect them for signs of breakage or abnormal wear before introducing them into a joint.

Skin or Urogenital Injury

Dermal burns sustained during hip arthroscopy are uncommon. Curtin and Friebe[17] reported a case in which irrigation fluid heated by a radiofrequency wand caused a second-degree burn when the outflow valve was left open to drain onto the patient's lateral thigh. This appears to be the only case report of a dermal burn after hip arthroscopy, although similar complications have been reported during shoulder or knee arthroscopy.[18,19] Although most studies of fluid temperature during arthroscopy focus on capsular tissue damage or chondrolysis, these case reports of dermal burns illustrate the importance of conscientious fluid management and monitoring for fluid leaks during arthroscopic procedures.

Urogenital injury is also an uncommon complication of hip arthroscopy. Clarke and colleagues[2] report only 1 such event among 1054 consecutive hip arthroscopies. Both the supine and lateral positions for hip arthroscopy put the patient at risk of sustaining such an injury due to the location of the perineal post. Poor patient positioning or a perineal post that is not adequately padded can lead to injuries such as scrotal pressure wounds, labia hematomas, or vaginal lacerations.[2,20,21] It is important for surgeons to use the minimal force and duration of traction that is needed to safely and adequately complete the hip arthroscopy. Similarly, before draping out the operative site, the surgeon should confirm the patient is safely and appropriately positioned. In males, genital crush injury is a significant risk if caution is not exercised during positioning and traction application.

Heterotopic Ossification

Heterotopic ossification (HO) is an osteogenic response within soft tissue that leads to ectopic bone formation often following trauma, surgery, burns, and neurologic injuries.[22] In cases in which a small foci of bone develops within a large muscle, HO may be asymptomatic or an incidental radiographic finding; however, when a larger mass of HO develops around a joint, it can lead to discomfort or loss of motion. HO is most commonly classified according to the criteria described by Brooker and colleagues[23] (**Table 1**).

For clinical situations in which there is a high risk of HO, prophylactic treatment using nonsteroidal anti-inflammatory drugs (NSAIDs) or radiation is often recommended. Numerous studies have found no difference between the 2 for the prevention of HO, and prophylaxis strategies must be determined on an individual basis.[22] The ideal NSAID, dose, and duration remain unclear for inhibiting ectopic bone formation while minimizing side effects.

The prevalence of HO can vary from less than 1% to 90% depending on the inciting etiology.[22] In patients not receiving prophylaxis, the incidence of HO following hip arthroscopy has been reported to be as high as 33% and 44% in 2 studies[24,25] (**Fig. 2**). Postoperative HO also has been reported in hip arthroscopy portal sites.[26] A cohort study by Beckmann and colleagues[27] found an incidence of 25% (23/92) in patients after hip arthroscopy who did not receive NSAID prophylaxis, compared with 5.6% (11/196) among patients who had taken naproxen 500 mg twice daily for 3 weeks starting on the first postoperative day. Patients who did not receive prophylaxis were 13.6 times more likely to develop postoperative HO. On multivariate logistic regression, the investigators found that in addition to the absence of NSAID prophylaxis, HO development was also predicted by resection of mixed-type femoroacetabular impingement (FAI) compared with either femoral osteochondroplasty or acetabuloplasty alone. All 34 cases of HO occurred anterior to the hip joint, and 9 were symptomatic enough to warrant surgical resection.

A cohort study by Bedi and colleagues[28] found a 4.7% (29/616) incidence of HO following hip arthroscopy. There was a statistically significant difference in the development of HO between patients who received prophylaxis with naproxen and indomethacin (1.8%) versus those who received naproxen alone (8.3%). Among the 29 cases of HO, 14 occurred anterior and 15 occurred lateral to the hip joint. In all 7 patients whose symptoms necessitated HO excision, the HO was located anterior to the hip joint. The investigators stress that it is important to correlate any postoperative symptoms with the location of the HO before proceeding with surgical excision.

Table 1	
Brooker classification system for hip heterotopic ossification	
Class	**Description**
I	Islands of bone within the soft tissues about the hip
II	Bone spurs from the pelvis or proximal end of the femur, leaving at least 1 cm between opposing bone surfaces
III	Bone spurs from the pelvis or proximal end of the femur, reducing the space between opposing bone surfaces to <1 cm
IV	Apparent bone ankylosis of the hip

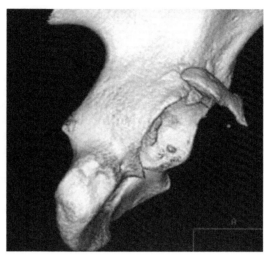

Fig. 2. Following right hip arthroscopic surgery, HO developed in the gluteus minimus musculature. This was treated nonoperatively, as there were no functional limitations.

Abdominal Compartment Syndrome

Intra-abdominal fluid extravasation (IAFE), intra-abdominal hypertension (IAH), and abdominal compartment syndrome (ACS) are rare complications of hip arthroscopy but are complications that may result in high morbidity and mortality. A survey of expert hip arthroscopists found 40 cases of IAFE among 25,648 hip arthroscopies (0.16% prevalence) with statistically significant risk factors, including higher arthroscopic fluid pump pressure and concomitant iliopsoas tenotomy.[29] Bartlett and colleagues[30] reported the first case of IAFE after hip arthroscopy for intra-articular loose body removal following open reduction and internal fixation of an acetabular fracture. The investigators hypothesized that arthroscopic fluid extravasation occurred through the fracture site, resulting in IAFE and eventually cardiac arrest. In other cases not involving acetabular fractures, investigators hypothesize that irrigation fluid follows a retroperitoneal course along the iliopsoas and iliac vessels, ultimately reaching the abdominal cavity via a disruption within the peritoneum.[31–33] To reduce the duration of time over which fluid extravasation may occur, it is recommended that iliopsoas tenotomy be performed toward the end of the case.

The World Society on Abdominal Compartment Syndrome has published consensus documents on the definitions, classification, diagnosis, and management of IAH and ACS.[34] The diagnosis of IAH/ACS is made by serial physical examination, careful monitoring of hemodynamic status, intra-abdominal pressure measurement, and abdominal imaging with ultrasound or computed tomography. The first signs or symptoms of IAH/ACS may include abdominal pain, abdominal distension, degradation of vital signs (hypothermia, bradycardia, hypotension), increased respiratory effort, unresponsiveness, metabolic acidosis, and elevated bladder or intra-abdominal pressures. Abdominal distension and pain may be difficult to assess intra-operatively due to the surgical drapes and the effects of anesthesia, respectively, so the surgeon must recognize other clues of fluid extravasation, such as inability to distend the joint, increased irrigation fluid requirements, pump irrigation system pressure sensor warnings, and increased thigh distension.

If left untreated, IAH/ACS can progress toward profound hemodynamic instability, compromised end-organ function, organ failure, or death. Treatment strategies depend on the etiology of the IAH/ACS and the clinical condition of the patient. The ultimate goal of treatment is to optimize systemic perfusion and organ function while addressing the underlying cause via medical or surgical interventions. There should be a low threshold for obtaining a general surgical consultation. Appropriate treatments may include observation, body positioning, sedation and analgesia, nasogastric decompression, fluid resuscitation, diuretics, renal replacement therapy, image-guided paracentesis and drainage, or open abdominal decompression.[34] Although abdominal decompression immediately reduces intra-abdominal pressure and can be life-saving, the morbidity of the procedure is warranted only when the condition is refractory to noninvasive treatment options.

PITFALLS TO AVOID AND TIPS FOR A SUCCESSFUL HIP ARTHROSCOPY
Learning Curve

Multiple studies have demonstrated that complication rates decrease with experience, and, unfortunately, this may be a nonmodifiable risk factor.[4,5,35–37] For FAI, a frequent reason for reoperation is incomplete correction of the osseous deformities, and improved ability to access and instrument these lesions is likely gained with experience[4,38] (**Fig. 3**). After 40 consecutive patients and a 20% failure rate, Lee and colleagues[36] used a cumulative sum analysis to estimate that 20 cases are required to achieve consistent clinical outcomes. Conversely, a retrospective series of 194 patients demonstrated that although the number of complications did not change with experience, the type of complication did.[5] Hoppe and colleagues[37] performed a systematic review examining the learning curve, and although after 30 cases there appeared to be a reduction in complications and operative time, they were hesitant to use a number to quantify the curve for all surgeons. Although most surgeons agree that a steep learning curve does exist, there is likely large variability among surgeons as to how many cases are required before they become proficient at hip arthroscopy and are able to thoroughly address more challenging deformities.

Asymptomatic Radiographic Findings

Although patients with FAI frequently present with intermittent, activity-related groin pain, FAI morphology among asymptomatic adults and adolescents is not

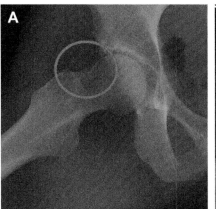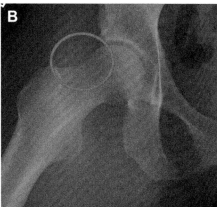

Fig. 3. Frog-leg lateral radiographs of the right hip (A) after incomplete arthroscopic resection of a cam impingement lesion (*highlighted area*) and (B) after revision resection demonstrating appropriate bony contour of the femoral neck.

uncommon.[39–42] Using MRI, Hack and colleagues[40] identified at least one hip with cam morphology in 14% of 200 asymptomatic volunteers. Jung and colleagues[41] used computed tomography scans to measure α-angles in asymptomatic adults. Hips were defined as borderline in 14.88% of men and 6.11% of women and pathologic in 13.95% of men and 5.56% of women. A systematic review by Frank and colleagues[39] included 2114 asymptomatic hips and demonstrated a 37.0% prevalence of cam deformity, 67.0% prevalence of pincer deformity, and 68.1% prevalence of labral injury on MRI without intra-articular contrast (although only 7 studies reported on labral injury). In other words, FAI is a clinical, rather than radiographic, diagnosis.

It has become increasingly recognized that some patients who have poor outcomes after hip arthroscopy may have additional pathology or have an incorrect diagnosis. The hip is a complex joint, and patients may have compensatory pain from surrounding structures, which may confuse the diagnosis.[43] For example, athletic pubalgia is commonly seen in patients with FAI, and a thorough physical examination must be performed to rule in or out concomitant pathologies.[44] Given the broad differential diagnosis for hip and groin pain, it is imperative that surgeons correlate history and physical examination with symptoms to avoid operating on patients with asymptomatic findings on imaging studies.

Osteoarthritis

Many studies have identified joint space narrowing and osteoarthritis as negative predictors of good clinical outcomes following hip arthroscopy with high rates of conversion to total hip arthroplasty (THA)[45–51] (**Fig. 4**). Larson and colleagues[45] found that failure rates following arthroscopic treatment of FAI were 12% in patients with FAI alone, 33% in patients with FAI and mild to moderate preoperative joint space narrowing (<50% joint space narrowing or >2 mm joint space), and 82% in patients with FAI and advanced preoperative joint space narrowing (>50% joint space narrowing or ≤2 mm joint space). Patients with advanced preoperative joint space narrowing did

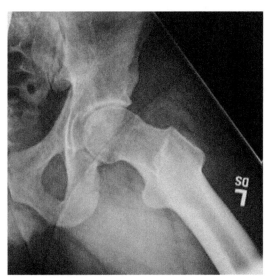

Fig. 4. Frog-leg lateral radiograph of the left hip shows mild osteoarthritis of the acetabular dome and lateral acetabular margin. Although these findings are mild, this patient would be at risk for postoperative failure of hip arthroscopy and for conversion to a THA.

not show clinical improvement at any time during the course of the study. These findings are consistent with other studies that identify ≤2 mm of joint space as contributing to suboptimal outcomes following arthroscopic hip procedures.[46,47] A systematic review of complications and reoperations following hip arthroscopy identified THA as the most common reason for reoperation (2.9%).[51] Using THA as an endpoint, McCarthy and colleagues[50] found that 10-year survivorship following hip arthroscopy was 80% in patients with lower Outerbridge grades (0, I, II) compared with 12% to 20% survivorship for patients with higher Outerbridge grades (III, IV) depending on the location of the cartilage degeneration. Overall, patients with a higher grade of osteoarthritis were 20 to 60 times more likely to require THA. Among 20 patients with intraoperatively diagnosed cartilage lesions of Outerbridge II or greater, Horisberger and colleagues[49] found that at an average of 3 years following arthroscopic surgery for FAI, 50% of patients had or were planning on THA. Bogunovic and colleagues[48] identified 58 patients (60 hips) with a history of failed hip arthroscopy and found 22 hips with moderate to severe osteoarthritis requiring arthroplasty at a mean duration of only 31.6 months. The investigators concluded that in the setting of moderate to severe osteoarthritis, there was limited benefit to arthroscopy and recommended nonoperative management until arthroplasty.

Bony Morphology Not Amenable to Arthroscopic Treatment

Hip arthroscopy may have a more limited application in certain types of bony morphology such as hip dysplasia, coxa profunda, protrusio acetabuli, femoral neck retroversion, femoral neck offset, and relative acetabular retroversion with decreased posterior coverage (**Fig. 5**). Addressing these conditions arthroscopically requires great technical expertise and concerns remain regarding the ability to adequately access and correct such deformities.[52–54] For example, in cases of protrusio acetabuli, the deformity may include medial acetabular dysplasia and relative neck shortening, neither of which would be addressed arthroscopically.[55,56] In such cases of complex deformity, techniques such as open surgical dislocation or anteverting periacetabular osteotomy may be more appropriate.[35]

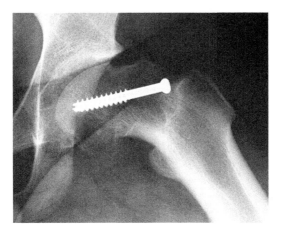

Fig. 5. Frog-leg lateral radiograph demonstrating a prior slipped capital femoral epiphysis with resulting femoral head retroversion, decreased femoral neck offset, abnormal head tilt, and cam-type morphology. This patient's pathology would not be correctable with arthroscopic decompression alone.

Hip Destabilization

Hip joint stability relies on osseous anatomy, the acetabular labrum, and the ligamentous hip capsule. Deficiency of these structures can result in instability, pain, and functional limitations. The acetabular labrum is important for maintaining hip stability, joint fluid seal, and intra-articular lubrication and fluid pressure, which help protect articular cartilage.[57–59] Hip capsule management, including both the longitudinal external fibers (iliofemoral, ischiofemoral, and pubofemoral ligaments) and the internal circumferential fibers (zona orbicularis), is critical for maintaining the stability and kinematics of the hip joint.[60,61] The literature comparing complete capsular repair versus partial repair or nonrepair is limited and additional long-term studies are needed.[62,63]

Hip instability following arthroscopy has been reported in the literature. Matsuda reported a patient who had anterior hip dislocation in the recovery room following capsulotomy and partial capsulectomy, mixed-type FAI resection, and labral debridement due to unsuccessful attempts at refixation.[64] The hip remained grossly unstable despite multiple closed reductions and bracing. The patient was subsequently treated with mini-open capsular repair. Following this experience, the investigator revised his labral refixation technique to minimize suture cut-through and advocated minimization of capsular disruption and selective arthroscopic capsular repair. Case reports of similar experiences involve patients with underlying conditions that predispose to hip instability, such as hip dysplasia and generalized ligamentous laxity; however, they still stress the importance of maintaining the labrum and capsule to optimize postoperative hip stability[65,66] (**Fig. 6**). It is particularly important to be cognizant that patients with acetabular retroversion with posterior undercoverage or subspine impingement may present with similar clinical and radiographic findings as patients with pincer-type FAI; however, in such patients arthroscopic resection of the anterior acetabulum may precipitate iatrogenic global undercoverage and hip instability.[67,68]

Obesity

The detrimental effects of obesity on various orthopedic conditions and outcomes are well studied; however, the literature on obesity as it relates to hip arthroscopy is less extensive. Collins and colleagues[69] compared obese and nonobese groups in patient-reported outcomes and complications following hip arthroscopy. Both

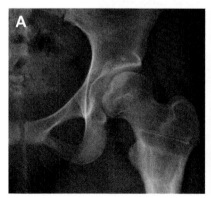 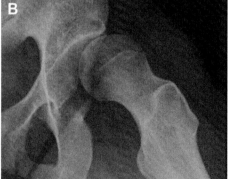

Fig. 6. (*A*) A preoperative anteroposterior radiograph of the left hip demonstrating hip dysplasia. (*B*) After arthroscopic hip surgery and capsulotomy without closure, the hip developed iatrogenic instability and lateralization of the femur.

groups had similar traction times, operative times, and improved clinical outcomes; however, obese patients were at 11.1 times greater odds for developing a postoperative complication. After 680 primary hip arthroscopies, Gupta and colleagues[70] noted that, although obese patients had lower absolute baseline and postoperative outcomes scores, the postoperative improvement among the obese cohort was not significantly different from the nonobese group. Limitations of these studies include relatively small sample sizes, inclusion of various arthroscopic procedures, and lack of long-term follow-up. As obesity has been shown to be a significant predictor of suboptimal outcomes in various orthopedic subspecialties, including lower extremity arthroplasty, trauma, and spine and knee arthroscopy, additional high-quality long-term studies are needed to understand the effects of obesity following hip arthroscopy.

Surgical Technique

Numerous studies have identified that incomplete surgical correction of FAI with residual osseous deformity is the primary cause for revision hip arthroscopy.[48,71,72] Philippon and colleagues[72] reported that among 37 patients having revision hip arthroscopy, 36 had radiographic evidence of unaddressed or inadequately addressed FAI, and 34 reported that their symptoms had not resolved after previous arthroscopy. Revision procedures were for residual FAI (95%), labral lesions (87%), chondral defects (70%), lysis of adhesions (63%), and previously unaddressed instability (35%). Similarly, Heyworth and colleagues[73] found that 54% of patients experienced no significant symptomatic improvement after initial arthroscopy and 79% had untreated or undertreated FAI lesions. In 2015, 2 systematic reviews of revision hip arthroscopy found that residual FAI was the most common indication for surgery.[38,74] When the surgeon believes bony resection is complete, a thorough evaluation should be performed to assess for residual impingement. Dynamic hip range of motion should assess for residual impingement in extension, abduction, internal rotation, external rotation, FABER (maximum flexion, abduction, external rotation), and FADIR (maximum flexion, adduction, internal rotation). Motion in these planes should be compared with preoperative measurements. Intraoperative fluoroscopic evaluation should include anteroposterior, cross-table lateral, 45° and 90° Dunn lateral views to confirm improved acetabular morphology, and "around-the-world" views to confirm normal head-neck junction and femoral head sphericity. These images should be compared with preoperative imaging studies. Ross and colleagues[75] described 6 critical fluoroscopic images to assess the most common zones of proximal femoral deformity and ensure thorough correction.

SUMMARY

Although hip arthroscopy continues to increase in popularity as the indications expand and surgeons become more comfortable with the techniques and instrumentation, the complications from this procedure can contribute to poor outcomes. A combination of careful preoperative planning with meticulous attention to sound intraoperative technique is critical to reduce risk of complications and failures.

REFERENCES

1. Sing DC, Feeley BT, Tay B, et al. Age-related trends in hip arthroscopy: a large cross-sectional analysis. Arthroscopy 2015;31(12):2307–13.e2.
2. Clarke MT, Arora A, Villar RN. Hip arthroscopy: complications in 1054 cases. Clin Orthop Relat Res 2003;(406):84–8.

3. Kowalczuk M, Bhandari M, Farrokhyar F, et al. Complications following hip arthroscopy: a systematic review and meta-analysis. Knee Surg Sports Traumatol Arthrosc 2013;21(7):1669–75.

4. Gupta A, Redmond JM, Hammarstedt JE, et al. Safety measures in hip arthroscopy and their efficacy in minimizing complications: a systematic review of the evidence. Arthroscopy 2014;30(10):1342–8.

5. Souza BG, Dani WS, Honda EK, et al. Do complications in hip arthroscopy change with experience? Arthroscopy 2010;26(8):1053–7.

6. Pailhé R, Chiron P, Reina N, et al. Pudendal nerve neuralgia after hip arthroscopy: retrospective study and literature review. Orthop Traumatol Surg Res 2013;99(7): 785–90.

7. Dippmann C, Thorborg K, Kraemer O, et al. Symptoms of nerve dysfunction after hip arthroscopy: an under-reported complication? Arthroscopy 2014;30(2): 202–7.

8. Merrell G, Medvecky M, Daigneault J, et al. Hip arthroscopy without a perineal post: a safer technique for hip distraction. Arthroscopy 2007;23(1):107.e1–3.

9. Byrd JW, Pappas JN, Pedley MJ. Hip arthroscopy: an anatomic study of portal placement and relationship to the extra-articular structures. Arthroscopy 1995; 11(4):418–23.

10. Watson JN, Bohnenkamp F, El-Bitar Y, et al. Variability in locations of hip neurovascular structures and their proximity to hip arthroscopic portals. Arthroscopy 2014;30(4):462–7.

11. Grothaus MC, Holt M, Mekhail AO, et al. Lateral femoral cutaneous nerve: an anatomic study. Clin Orthop Relat Res 2005;(437):164–8.

12. Thorey F, Ezechieli M, Ettinger M, et al. Access to the hip joint from standard arthroscopic portals: a cadaveric study. Arthroscopy 2013;29(8):1297–307.

13. Badylak JS, Keene JS. Do iatrogenic punctures of the labrum affect the clinical results of hip arthroscopy? Arthroscopy 2011;27(6):761–7.

14. Domb B, Hanypsiak B, Botser I. Labral penetration rate in a consecutive series of 300 hip arthroscopies. Am J Sports Med 2012;40(4):864–9.

15. Aoki SK, Beckmann JT, Wylie JD. Hip arthroscopy and the anterolateral portal: avoiding labral penetration and femoral articular injuries. Arthrosc Tech 2012; 1(2):e155–60.

16. Nwachukwu BU, McFeely ED, Nasreddine AY, et al. Complications of hip arthroscopy in children and adolescents. J Pediatr Orthop 2011;31(3):227–31.

17. Curtin B, Friebe I. Dermal burn during hip arthroscopy. Orthopedics 2014;37(8): e746–9.

18. Kouk SN, Zoric B, Stetson WB. Complication of the use of a radiofrequency device in arthroscopic shoulder surgery: second-degree burn of the shoulder girdle. Arthroscopy 2011;27(1):136–41.

19. Huang S, Gateley D, Moss AL. Accidental burn injury during knee arthroscopy. Arthroscopy 2007;23(12):1363.e1–3.

20. Funke EL, Munzinger U. Complications in hip arthroscopy. Arthroscopy 1996; 12(2):156–9.

21. Eriksson E, Arvidsson I, Arvidsson H. Diagnostic and operative arthroscopy of the hip. Orthopedics 1986;9(2):169–76.

22. Ranganathan K, Loder S, Agarwal S, et al. Heterotopic ossification: basic-science principles and clinical correlates. J Bone Joint Surg Am 2015;97(13): 1101–11.

23. Brooker AF, Bowerman JW, Robinson RA, et al. Ectopic ossification following total hip replacement. Incidence and a method of classification. J Bone Joint Surg Am 1973;55(8):1629–32.
24. Rath E, Sherman H, Sampson TG, et al. The incidence of heterotopic ossification in hip arthroscopy. Arthroscopy 2013;29(3):427–33.
25. Randelli F, Pierannunzii L, Banci L, et al. Heterotopic ossifications after arthroscopic management of femoroacetabular impingement: the role of NSAID prophylaxis. J Orthop Traumatol 2010;11(4):245–50.
26. Ozturk BY, Kelly BT. Heterotopic ossification in portal sites following hip arthroscopy. Arch Orthop Trauma Surg 2013;133(7):979–84.
27. Beckmann JT, Wylie JD, Kapron AL, et al. The effect of NSAID prophylaxis and operative variables on heterotopic ossification after hip arthroscopy. Am J Sports Med 2014;42(6):1359–64.
28. Bedi A, Zbeda RM, Bueno VF, et al. The incidence of heterotopic ossification after hip arthroscopy. Am J Sports Med 2012;40(4):854–63.
29. Kocher MS, Frank JS, Nasreddine AY, et al. Intra-abdominal fluid extravasation during hip arthroscopy: a survey of the MAHORN group. Arthroscopy 2012;28(11):1654–60.e2.
30. Bartlett CS, DiFelice GS, Buly RL, et al. Cardiac arrest as a result of intraabdominal extravasation of fluid during arthroscopic removal of a loose body from the hip joint of a patient with an acetabular fracture. J Orthop Trauma 1998;12(4):294–9.
31. Fowler J, Owens BD. Abdominal compartment syndrome after hip arthroscopy. Arthroscopy 2010;26(1):128–30.
32. Verma M, Sekiya JK. Intrathoracic fluid extravasation after hip arthroscopy. Arthroscopy 2010;26(9):S90–4.
33. Haupt U, Volkle D, Waldherr C, et al. Intra- and retroperitoneal irrigation liquid after arthroscopy of the hip joint. Arthroscopy 2008;24(8):966–8.
34. Cheatham ML, Malbrain ML, Kirkpatrick A, et al. Results from the international conference of experts on intra-abdominal hypertension and abdominal compartment syndrome. II. Recommendations. Intensive Care Med 2007;33(6):951–62.
35. Zaltz I, Kelly BT, Larson CM, et al. Surgical treatment of femoroacetabular impingement: what are the limits of hip arthroscopy? Arthroscopy 2014;30(1):99–110.
36. Lee YK, Ha YC, Hwang DS, et al. Learning curve of basic hip arthroscopy technique: CUSUM analysis. Knee Surg Sports Traumatol Arthrosc 2013;21(8):1940–4.
37. Hoppe DJ, de Sa D, Simunovic N, et al. The learning curve for hip arthroscopy: a systematic review. Arthroscopy 2014;30(3):389–97.
38. Sardana V, Philippon MJ, de Sa D, et al. Revision hip arthroscopy indications and outcomes: a systematic review. Arthroscopy 2015;31(10):2047–55.
39. Frank JM, Harris JD, Erickson BJ, et al. Prevalence of femoroacetabular impingement imaging findings in asymptomatic volunteers: a systematic review. Arthroscopy 2015;31(6):1199–204.
40. Hack K, Di Primio G, Rakhra K, et al. Prevalence of cam-type femoroacetabular impingement morphology in asymptomatic volunteers. J Bone Joint Surg Am 2010;92(14):2436–44.
41. Jung KA, Restrepo C, Hellman M, et al. The prevalence of cam-type femoroacetabular deformity in asymptomatic adults. J Bone Joint Surg Br 2011;93(10):1303–7.

42. Li Y, Helvie P, Mead M, et al. Prevalence of femoroacetabular impingement morphology in asymptomatic adolescents. J Pediatr Orthop 2015. [Epub ahead of print].

43. Bedi A, Dolan M, Leunig M, et al. Static and dynamic mechanical causes of hip pain. Arthroscopy 2011;27(2):235–51.

44. Hammoud S, Bedi A, Magennis E, et al. High incidence of athletic pubalgia symptoms in professional athletes with symptomatic femoroacetabular impingement. Arthroscopy 2012;28(10):1388–95.

45. Larson CM, Giveans MR, Taylor M. Does arthroscopic FAI correction improve function with radiographic arthritis? Clin Orthop Relat Res 2011;469:1667–76.

46. Ayeni OR, Alradwan H, de Sa D, et al. The hip labrum reconstruction: indications and outcomes–a systematic review. Knee Surg Sports Traumatol Arthrosc 2014; 22(4):737–43.

47. Philippon MJ, Briggs KK, Carlisle JC, et al. Joint space predicts THA after hip arthroscopy in patients 50 years and older. Clin Orthop Relat Res 2013;471(8): 2492–6.

48. Bogunovic L, Gottlieb M, Pashos G, et al. Why do hip arthroscopy procedures fail? Clin Orthop Relat Res 2013;471(8):2523–9.

49. Horisberger M, Brunner A, Herzog RF. Arthroscopic treatment of femoral acetabular impingement in patients with preoperative generalized degenerative changes. Arthroscopy 2010;26(5):623–9.

50. McCarthy JC, Jarrett BT, Ojeifo O, et al. What factors influence long-term survivorship after hip arthroscopy? Clin Orthop Relat Res 2011;469(2):362–71.

51. Harris JD, McCormick FM, Abrams GD, et al. Complications and reoperations during and after hip arthroscopy: a systematic review of 92 studies and more than 6,000 patients. Arthroscopy 2013;29(3):589–95.

52. Matsuda DK. Protrusio acetabuli: contraindication or indication for hip arthroscopy? And the case for arthroscopic treatment of global pincer impingement. Arthroscopy 2012;28(6):882–8.

53. Safran MR, Epstein NP. Arthroscopic management of protrusio acetabuli. Arthroscopy 2013;29(11):1777–82.

54. Matsuda DK, Gupta N, Hanami D. Hip arthroscopy for challenging deformities: global pincer femoroacetabular impingement. Arthrosc Tech 2014;3(2):e197–204.

55. Liechti EF, Ferguson SJ, Tannast M. Protrusio acetabuli: joint loading with severe pincer impingement and its theoretical implications for surgical therapy. J Orthop Res 2014;33(1):106–13.

56. Leunig M, Nho SJ, Turchetto L, et al. Protrusio acetabuli: new insights and experience with joint preservation. Clin Orthop Relat Res 2009;467(9):2241–50.

57. Cadet ER, Chan AK, Vorys GC, et al. Investigation of the preservation of the fluid seal effect in the repaired, partially resected, and reconstructed acetabular labrum in a cadaveric hip model. Am J Sports Med 2012;40(10):2218–23.

58. Crawford MJ, Dy CJ, Alexander JW, et al. The biomechanics of the hip labrum and the stability of the hip. Clin Orthop Relat Res 2007;465:16–22.

59. Smith MV, Panchal HB, Ruberte Thiele RA, et al. Effect of acetabular labrum tears on hip stability and labral strain in a joint compression model. Am J Sports Med 2011;39:103S–10S.

60. Bedi A, Galano G, Walsh C, et al. Capsular management during hip arthroscopy: from femoroacetabular impingement to instability. Arthroscopy 2011;27(12): 1720–31.

61. Smith MV, Sekiya JK. Hip instability. Sports Med Arthrosc 2010;18(2):108–12.

62. Domb BG, Stake CE, Finley ZJ, et al. Influence of capsular repair versus unrepaired capsulotomy on 2-year clinical outcomes after arthroscopic hip preservation surgery. Arthroscopy 2015;31(4):643–50.

63. Frank RM, Lee S, Bush-Joseph C, et al. Improved outcomes after hip arthroscopic surgery in patients undergoing T-capsulotomy with complete repair versus partial repair for femoroacetabular impingement: a comparative matched-pair analysis. Am J Sports Med 2014;42(11):2634–42.

64. Matsuda DK. Acute iatrogenic dislocation following hip impingement arthroscopic surgery. Arthroscopy 2009;25(4):400–4.

65. Benali Y, Katthagen BD. Hip subluxation as a complication of arthroscopic debridement. Arthroscopy 2009;25(4):405–7.

66. Ranawat AS, McClincy M, Sekiya JK. Anterior dislocation of the hip after arthroscopy in a patient with capsular laxity of the hip. A case report. J Bone Joint Surg Am 2009;91(1):192–7.

67. Larson CM, Kelly BT, Stone RM. Making a case for anterior inferior iliac spine/subspine hip impingement: three representative case reports and proposed concept. Arthroscopy 2011;27(12):1732–7.

68. Zaltz I, Kelly BT, Hetsroni I, et al. The crossover sign overestimates acetabular retroversion. Clin Orthop Relat Res 2013;471(8):2463–70.

69. Collins JA, Beutel BG, Garofolo G, et al. Correlation of obesity with patient-reported outcomes and complications after hip arthroscopy. Arthroscopy 2015;31(1):57–62.

70. Gupta A, Redmond JM, Hammarstedt JE, et al. Does obesity affect outcomes in hip arthroscopy? A matched-pair controlled study with minimum 2-year follow-up. Am J Sports Med 2015;43(4):965–71.

71. Clohisy JC, Nepple JJ, Larson CM, et al. Persistent structural disease is the most common cause of repeat hip preservation surgery. Clin Orthop Relat Res 2013;471(12):3788–94.

72. Philippon MJ, Schenker ML, Briggs KK, et al. Revision hip arthroscopy. Am J Sports Med 2007;35(11):1918–21.

73. Heyworth BE, Shindle MK, Voos JE, et al. Radiologic and intraoperative findings in revision hip arthroscopy. Arthroscopy 2007;23(12):1295–302.

74. Cvetanovich GL, Harris JD, Erickson BJ, et al. Revision hip arthroscopy: a systematic review of diagnoses, operative findings, and outcomes. Arthroscopy 2015;31(7):1382–90.

75. Ross JR, Bedi A, Stone RM, et al. Intraoperative fluoroscopic imaging to treat cam deformities: correlation with 3-dimensional computed tomography. Am J Sports Med 2014;42(6):1370–6.

Rehabilitation After Hip Arthroscopy

A Movement Control–Based Perspective

Philip Malloy, MS, PT, SCS[a],*, Kim Gray, DPT[b], Andrew B. Wolff, MD[c]

KEYWORDS

- Rehabilitation • Hip arthroscopy • Movement control • Hip rehabilitation

KEY POINTS

- Joint protection immediately after hip arthroscopy is essential and must be tailored specifically to the severity of hip injury and surgical procedures performed.
- Mobility, muscle performance and stability, and neuromuscular control are vital aspects to movement control that are commonly addressed in rehabilitation programs after hip arthroscopy.
- Each phase of hip arthroscopy should be adapted to the specific functional demands of the patient. Exercise progressions should be monitored closely and patients should be progressed slowly to prevent complications, such as persistent soft tissue irritation.

BACKGROUND

Diagnosis and management of nonarthritic hip pathology have evolved significantly over the years through the advancements in arthroscopic surgical interventions for intra-articular and extra-articular hip injury.[1] The rapid growth of hip arthroscopic surgery necessitates parallel advancement in rehabilitation after surgery.[2–4] Currently, much of the evidence on rehabilitation after hip arthroscopy is limited to case-control studies.[5–9] In part, this population is difficult to study because hip arthroscopy often requires patient-specific postoperative restrictions. Additionally, the diverse backgrounds of rehabilitation specialists creates a situation where different treatment techniques may be equally effective based on a patient's specific need.

In recent years, many investigators have presented guidelines for hip arthroscopy rehabilitation with much of the evidence based on empirical experience and rehabilitation literature from similar patient populations.[2–4,10,11] Most presented guidelines

Disclosures: Dr A.B. Wolff is a paid consultant for Strkyer.
^a Department of Physical Therapy, Marquette University, 604 North 16th Street, Milwaukee, WI 53233, USA; ^b SMARTherapy, Washington Orthopaedics and Sports Medicine, 2021 K Street Northwest, Washington, DC 20006, USA; ^c Department of Orthopedic Surgery, Washington Orthopaedics and Sports Medicine, 2021 K Street Northwest, Washington, DC 20006, USA
* Corresponding author.
E-mail address: Philip.malloy@marquette.edu

Clin Sports Med 35 (2016) 503–521
http://dx.doi.org/10.1016/j.csm.2016.02.012
0278-5919/16/$ – see front matter © 2016 Elsevier Inc. All rights reserved.

sportsmed.theclinics.com

break down hip arthroscopy rehabilitation into 4 or 5 phases. The focus of each phase is related to pivotal aspects of rehabilitation after surgery, which includes joint protection, range of motion and mobility, restoration of normal gait, muscle strength and neuromuscular control, and sport-specific or functional training.[2–4,11] Objective milestones for progression from one phase to the next provide clinicians and patients with tangible goals while respecting healing time frames for surgically repaired tissues.[12] In addition, many of these published guidelines provide surgery-specific limitations, for example, weight-bearing restriction after microfracture or range-of-motion limitation after soft tissue repair.[2,4,13] Other guidelines have presented pitfalls potentially encountered at each rehabilitative phase as well as prevention strategies to mitigate the occurrence of these setbacks.[3]

The understanding of human movement control is essential to the development of an effective rehabilitation program for patients after hip arthroscopy. Vital aspects of movement control include mobility, muscle performance and stability, and neuromuscular control, which serve as common rehabilitation targets for clinicians. Each of these aspects of movement control is essential for safe return to functional activities after hip arthroscopy. For that reason, it is the purpose of this article to present hip arthroscopy rehabilitation guidelines based on the important aspects of movement control. Initial joint protection techniques are discussed and rehabilitation is broken down into 4 phases in the context of mobility, muscle performance and stability, and neuromuscular control exercises.

JOINT PROTECTION

It is known that cellular repair and remodeling mechanisms begin immediately after joint injury or surgery.[14] To promote an optimal environment for healing, joint protection aimed at the restoration of joint homeostasis is the initial primary goal after hip arthroscopy. For practical purposes, joint homeostasis can be defined as the elimination of outward signs of acute or subacute inflammation, which may include edema, ecchymosis, pain at rest, and/or pain at the end of the day. Healing of the incision portal sites and a reduction in ecchymosis provides a good indication of when acute inflammation is no longer present. The rehabilitation during this phase is crucial to set the foundation for progression to the next phases. Emphasis should be placed on significant activity limitation and rest during this phase to allow the natural healing process to take place. Pharmacologic treatments during this phase include the use of pain medication and nonsteroidal anti-inflammatory drugs to reduce pain and inflammation and for prevention of heterotopic ossification after surgery.

Patient education on joint protection strategies is essential to prevent both intra-articular and extra-articular soft tissue irritation. Restricted weight bearing is commonly recommended to reduce joint reaction forces to protect healing tissues, such as the femoral neck, acetabular labrum, joint capsule, and contractile tissues of the hip joint.[15] Patients should be instructed in a foot flat or normal heel-toe weight-bearing pattern using an assistive device. The use of a non–weight-bearing or toe-touch weight-bearing pattern is contraindicated because this leads to recurrent activation of the hip flexor muscle group. Persistent activation of the hip flexors after surgery can result in persistent anterior pain secondary to muscle overuse. To prevent stiffness in the anterior hip during this initial phase, patients should be instructed to limit sitting time and encouraged to change positions frequently. Prone lying should be emphasized to position the hip in neutral; however, caution should be exercised for prone positioning in patients with low back pain.[13]

A continuous passive motion machine may be prescribed after surgery to begin controlled passive movement of the hip. Rehabilitation specialists must provide instruction on how to get in and out of the continuous passive motion machine to avoid actively lifting the leg immediately after surgery. In the first few postoperative days, caregiver assistance or the use of a leg-lifting device is helpful. Patients can begin riding an upright stationary bicycle the first week after surgery. Recumbent bicycles should be discouraged. Instructing patients on safe techniques for getting on and off a bike and setting the proper seat height to avoid pinching in the anterior hip is imperative.

MOBILITY
Phase 1 Mobility Exercises

Passive range-of-motion exercises can be initiated during the first week after hip arthroscopy. Although range-of-motion restrictions are procedure dependent, small oscillatory motions in the midranges of all planes are recommended.[16] Although cases of intra-articular adhesions have been reported, these complications are uncommon.[17,18] Therefore, during this phase, range-of-motion exercises should always be performed in pain-free ranges. In addition, limitation in specific motion, such as extension and external rotation, may be prescribed in patients where capsular modification or labral reconstruction procedures were performed.[2,12] The rehabilitation specialist must communicate with the surgeon to determine the extent of postoperative range-of-motion limitations on the tissues addressed.

Gentle soft tissue mobilization should be initiated in the first week postoperatively to assist with scar and edema management. Soft tissue mobilization may also be useful for pain reduction and increased tone in muscles surrounding the hip and trunk.[9]

Phase 2 Mobility Exercises

Passive range-of-motion exercises should be continued with gentle end-range stretching as needed. Active movements should be performed through larger arcs of motion and into terminal ranges while continuing to respect the surgery-specific range-of-motion restrictions. It may be useful for clinicians to use functional tests to assess range of motion into terminal ranges, such as a double-leg squat (**Fig. 1**) or standing hip hike (**Fig. 2**). Frontal plane mobility may be assessed with crossover stepping or a lateral slide side lunge (**Fig. 3**). A standing stool rotation exercise can be used to assess transverse plane hip mobility (**Fig. 4**). In patients with persistent mobility issues, soft tissue and joint mobilization may be beneficial. Prescribing a dynamic self-stretching program assists with maintaining the mobility gained with manual techniques. Also, performing active movements into the range of motion can assist with re-establishing movement control into the range.

Phase 3 Mobility Exercises

At this point, patients should have the required hip joint mobility for the desired functional activity. Using exercises to maintain this range of motion, however, especially as muscle size increases with training, is important. In addition, the ankle, knee, lumbar, and thoracic spine should be evaluated early in this phase to ensure adequate segmental mobility is present for advanced function and dynamic exercise. A dynamic warm-up or movement preparation exercises are recommended prior to a training session to ensure adequate warm-up and mobility before beginning exercise. Patients may return to yoga for stretching as long as the physician and therapist have released

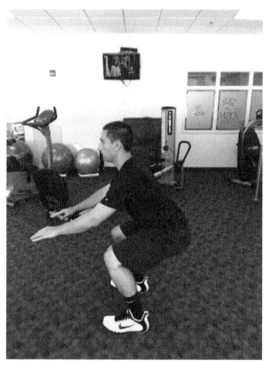

Fig. 1. Double-leg squat.

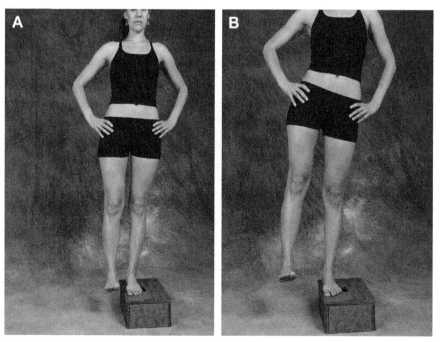

Fig. 2. (*A*) Standing and (*B*) hip hike. (*B*: *From* Malloy M, Wood R, Malloy P. Rehabilitation of non-operative hip conditions. In: Nho S, Leunig M, Larson M, et al, editors. Hip arthroscopy and hip joint preservation surgery. New York: Springer Science + Business Media, 2015; with permission.)

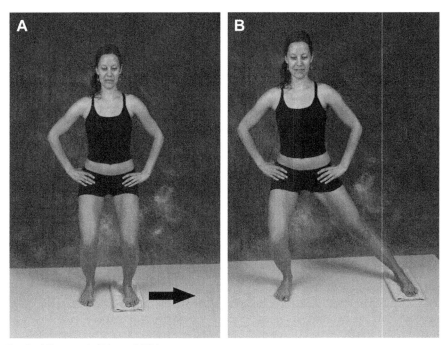

Fig. 3. (*A*) Lateral slide and (*B*) lunge.

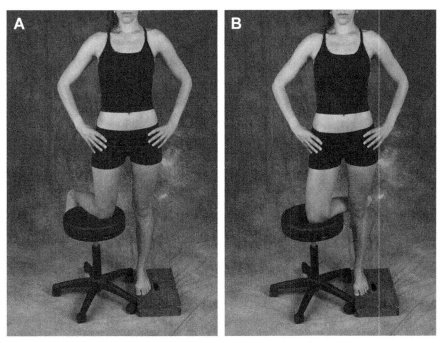

Fig. 4. Standing stool hip, (*A*) internal rotation and (*B*) external rotation.

the patient for this activity. Modifications of postures may be required, however, to prevent undue tissue stress.

MUSCLE PERFORMANCE AND STABILITY
Phase 1 Muscle Performance and Stability Exercises

Arthrogenic muscle inhibition of the gluteus maximus has been demonstrated in an experimental model of hip joint effusion.[19] Therefore, submaximal isometric exercises should be initiated early to reduce arthrogenic inhibition and other contributors to muscle atrophy, such as immobilization and disuse. The gluteus maximus, quadriceps, hamstrings, and abdominals should be the targets of initial isometric exercise, with instruction to avoid pain emphasized. Initial isometrics should be performed in different positions, such as prone and side lying.

Once muscle activation is established, patients can begin to perform simple movement patterns to facilitate muscle activation for stability. For example, previous investigators have noted the benefit of quadruped rocking (**Fig. 5**) for the restoration of hip flexion range of motion.[10,12,13] A simple abdominal brace helps maintain a neutral trunk and pelvis alignment during the movement. Small arc sagittal plane pelvic motion can also be performed in quadruped or a tall kneeling (**Fig. 6**) position to promote concentric muscle activation of the hip and trunk muscles. Upper extremity raises in quadruped can promote unilateral shoulder girdle muscle activation with simultaneous concentric activation of the raised upper extremity to begin to prepare for sequenced movements (**Fig. 7**).

Once initial muscle activation and stability are established, isolated strengthening exercises for the hip flexors, extensors, abductors, and adductors should be initiated to reduce weakness associated with surgery.[20] Initial isolated muscle exercises can include standing hip abductions (**Fig. 8**), neutral clamshells, and double-leg bridges. Double-leg standing, strengthening, and stability exercises can be performed with resistance band rows and latissimus pulldowns.

Phase 2 Muscle Performance and Stability Exercises

Muscle performance and stability must be progressed to meet the demands of gait and normal activities of daily living tasks during this phase 2. Modeling studies have shown isolated hip muscle weakness can lead to increased stress on the hip joint.[21] Therefore, foundational strength must be restored in phase 1 prior to progression to phase 2. To effectively address each aspect of muscle performance and stability in phase 2, therapists must alter the temporal and spatial variables of strengthening exercises. Timed isometric holds at multiple joint angles promote maximal strength

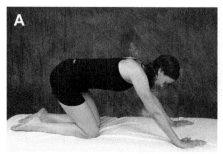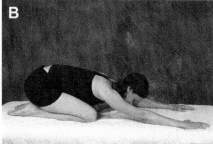

Fig. 5. (*A*) Quadruped and (*B*) rocking.

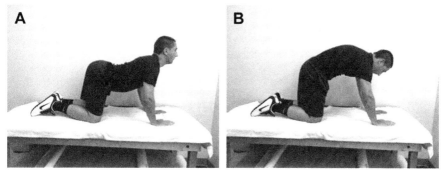

Fig. 6. (*A*) Anterior and (*B*) posterior pelvic tilt in quadruped.

through ranges of movement, and repeated concentric and eccentric muscle activations assist with patterning muscle recruitment during movement.[2] Muscle endurance can be improved by increasing the duration of activation in both types of exercise.

Single-leg balance exercises should be initiated early in this phase to prepare for single-limb stance during gait. Isometric hip abduction into a wall can is also useful to develop early hip abductor strength and can be progressed to single-leg stance with uninvolved isometric hip abduction for single-leg stance stability (**Fig. 9**). A single-leg bridge progression can help develop hip extensor strength, and standing double-leg slide board progressions can promote both eccentric and concentric muscle activation in isolated planes of motion (**Fig. 10**). Edelstein and colleagues[2] recommend seated posterior trunk leans (**Fig. 11**) to promote eccentric activation of the hip flexors, while proving manual cues to the hip adductor longus, rectus femoris, and tensor fascia lata muscles to prevent over-recruitment of these accessory hip flexors. The hip flexor muscle group primarily functions eccentrically during the stance phase of normal gait with a transition to concentric activation to initiate swing phase.[22] Simulation studies have demonstrated that gait is not as robust to weakness of the hip flexors compared with other sagittal plane hip muscle groups.[23] Therefore, it is essential to address hip flexor weakness and altered neuromuscular activation during this phase of hip arthroscopy rehabilitation. In addition, adequate trunk stability and muscle performance is fundamental to movement, such as normal gait. Forward (**Fig. 12**A–C) and side plank progression (**Fig. 13**A, B) have been shown effective in

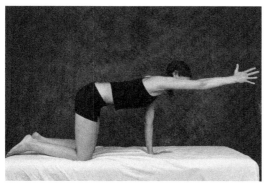

Fig. 7. Quadruped upper extremity raise.

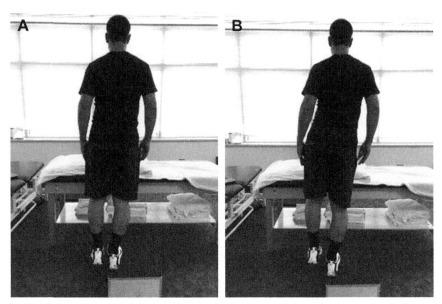

Fig. 8. (*A*) Standing and (*B*) hip abductions.

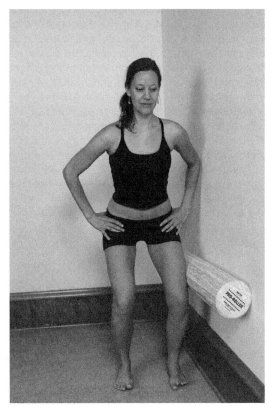

Fig. 9. Standing hip abduction isometric.

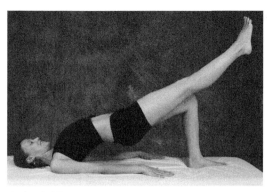

Fig. 10. Supine single-leg bridge.

achieving high levels of muscle activation of the core and trunk muscles; therefore, these common exercises should be initiated during this phase of hip arthroscopy rehabilitation.[24,25]

Phase 3 Muscle Performance and Stability Exercises

The ultimate goal of phase 3 hip arthroscopy rehabilitation is to return patients to unrestricted functional activities. The muscle performance and stability exercises during this phase are individual, based on a patient's specific functional demands. The therapist must initiate a clear discussion with patients about desired level of activity. Injury severity and consequences of the surgical procedures must be considered when

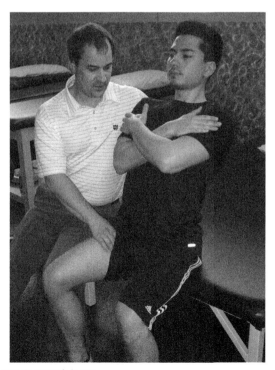

Fig. 11. Seated posterior trunk leans.

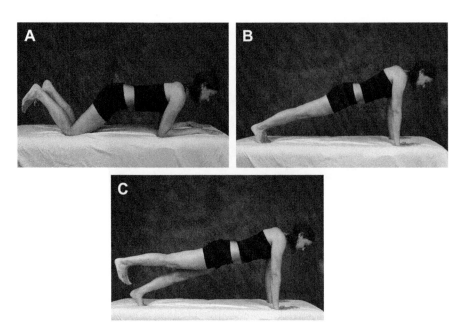

Fig. 12. Prone plank progression. (*A*) Modified on knee plank; (*B*) full plank; and (*C*) full plank with hip extension.

considering desired activity level. Realistic goals should be established with the purpose of long-term hip joint preservation, which, in some cases, may require modification of previous activity levels. It is vital for therapists to provide a comprehensive strengthening maintenance program that can be easily incorporated into a patient's normal exercise or daily routine so that the patient can sustain injury-free function.

In general, most muscle performance exercises during this phase involve the use of resistance or load to increase muscle strength. Single-leg squat progressions, which require both concentric and eccentric muscle activation, should begin in this phase. Initially, single-leg squats with balance support (**Fig. 14**) should be performed, progressing to unsupported single-leg squats (**Fig. 15**). Upper body strengthening exercise can be added during split-squat progressions to promote simultaneous trunk and upper body muscle activation, which is commonly encountered during functional tasks (**Fig. 16**). Often, muscle performance exercises in phase 3 incorporate aspects

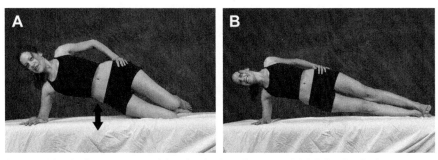

Fig. 13. Side plank progression. (*A*) Side plank on knees and (*B*) full side plank.

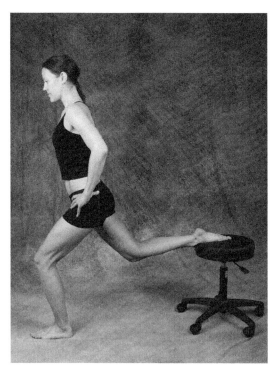

Fig. 14. Split balance squat. (*From* Malloy M, Wood R, Malloy P. Rehabilitation of non-operative hip conditions. In: Nho S, Leunig M, Larson M, et al, editors. Hip arthroscopy and hip joint preservation surgery. New York: Springer Science + Business Media, 2015; with permission.)

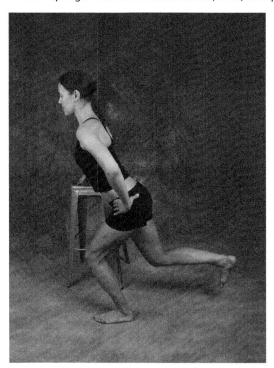

Fig. 15. Single-leg squat. (*From* Malloy M, Wood R, Malloy P. Rehabilitation of non-operative hip conditions. In: Nho S, Leunig M, Larson M, et al, editors. Hip arthroscopy and hip joint preservation surgery. New York: Springer Science + Business Media, 2015; with permission.)

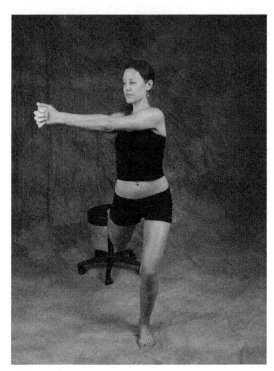

Fig. 16. Split squat with trunk rotation.

of neuromuscular control, such as coordination and sequencing. A single-leg squat exercise with a unilateral row requires appropriate muscle performance and segmental movement to maintain a neutral pelvic and trunk position during the movement (**Fig. 17**). In general, hip arthroscopy patients can be progressed during this phase as tolerated. Therapists are encouraged to use creativity when developing strengthening programs that uniquely meet the individual functional demands of the patient during this phase.

Phase 4 Muscle Performance and Stability Exercises

Muscle performance during the final phase of rehabilitation should focus on power development. Power is expressed as the product of force and velocity.[26] Muscle power output is dependent, however, on muscle length and type of activation performed. Although a full explanation of the mechanical variable of power is outside the scope of this article, clinicians should consider a few factors to improve power development for high-level activities in patients after hip arthroscopy. Muscles can produce the most power when a large force is produced at an intermediate velocity.[26] For example, when a person moves a heavy load that requires large force production at a relatively constant nonmaximal velocity, a large amount of power is produced during the movement as the muscles shorten. Conversely, a large amount of power can be produced if a large load is moved slowly as the muscle lengthens, as during an eccentric muscle activation phase of an activity. Therefore, muscle performance during this phase must focus on altering the variables of velocity and load to achieve the greatest amount of power output. In addition, therapists must consider whether the movement involves a concentric (shortening) or eccentric (lengthening) contraction of a muscle to appropriately alter the variables involved in power production.

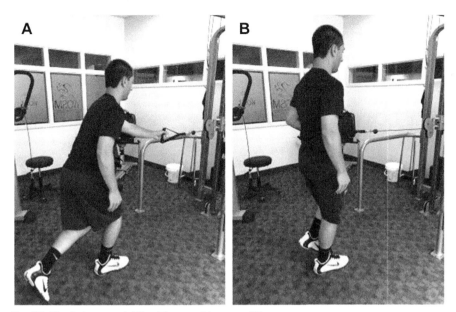

Fig. 17. Single leg squat (*A*) with a machine row (*B*).

NEUROMUSCULAR CONTROL
Phase 1 Neuromuscular Control Exercises

Initial neuromuscular control exercises should focus on appropriate muscle recruitment for smooth sequenced movements in isolated planes. A supine heel slide requires a sequenced activation of the abdominals to stabilize the pelvis and trunk while simultaneous activation of the hip flexors act to move the thigh. Aberrant motion (ie, out of sagittal plane deviation) of the thigh may indicate an alteration in muscle performance or activation timing. Supine bridging can be used to assess movement coordination that is essential for activities, such as transfers and bed mobility. In general, phase 1 neuromuscular control exercises look to identify and correct obvious aberrant (ie, out of plane) motion during basic activities of daily living. Additionally, posture should be evaluated with emphasis on neutral alignment during sitting and standing to prevent undue stress on healing hip joint tissue.

Phase 2 Neuromuscular Control Exercises

The focus of phase 2 is to re-establish coordination of movement patterns for gait, stair climbing, and other activities of daily living. As activity is advanced, appropriate movement sequencing must be achieved in hip arthroscopy patients so that undue stress in not placed on healing tissue. Initial exercises should involve single-plane movement patterns in ranges that are pain-free. Patients should begin exercises in half or tall kneeling positions to work on movement sequencing of the hip, pelvis, trunk, and upper extremities prior to a full weight-bearing position (**Fig. 18**).

Gait is one of a person's most basic functional requirements; therefore, the restoration of a normal gait pattern should be the primary focus of neuromuscular training phase 2. Tactile and visual feedback during exercise may assist patients in regaining aspects of proprioception that are affected by surgery. Manual techniques to promote muscle activation and facilitate pelvic and lower extremity motion are useful in helping restore normal gait (**Fig. 19**).

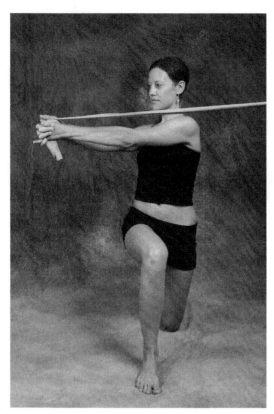

Fig. 18. Half-kneeling trunk rotations.

Individuals with symptomatic femoroacetabular impingement demonstrate movement pattern alterations both before and after corrective hip surgery during double-leg squats and a step-up task.[27–29] The double-leg squat is functional movement that serves as an excellent basis for neuromuscular training (see **Fig. 1**). Appropriate force development and transfer must be accomplished to successfully complete the exercise in neutral body alignment. Additionally, step-up and step-down exercises may be useful for evaluating neuromuscular control in this phase. Step-ups require neuromuscular control during predominantly concentric muscle activation whereas step-downs evaluate this control during eccentric activation demands. As a patient's neuromuscular control improves, additional planes of movement and simultaneous movement of other segments should be incorporated into the treatment program.

Phase 3 Neuromuscular Control Exercises

Neuromuscular control exercises during this phase must incorporate movement patterns that are consistent with an individual's function. Careful evaluation of movement timing during exercise to ensure appropriate force transfer during high-level functional tasks is indicated. Neuromuscular training in phase 3 should work to develop neuromuscular control as movement range, velocity, and load demands increase. Each of these movement variables must be tailored to patients' specific functional demands; therefore, this phase of rehabilitation is the most individualized.

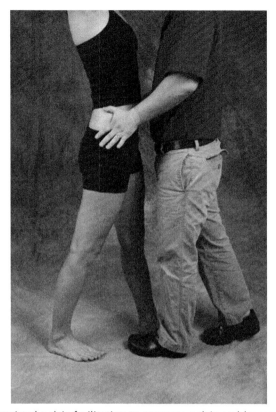

Fig. 19. Manual resisted pelvic facilitation to promote pelvic and lower extremity flexion during gait.

Exercise progressions during this phase blend aspects of muscle performance and neuromuscular control. Many progressions involve maintaining stability of one segment while another is moved. An example of this occurs during a side plank where the top leg can be flexed and extended to mimic a running type movement pattern. A wall lean with rapid high knee exercise can be used to sequence the rapid hip flexion needed to run. This exercise can be progressed to a high-box step-up to increase concentric demand on the stance leg during the movement.

Double-leg squat exercises can be progressed to incorporate simultaneous upper extremity pressing to assist with force transfer between the upper body and lower body. Single-leg stance with rapid stepping with a resistance band around patients' ankles promotes both stability and neuromuscular control of each limb simultaneously, which is often required in higher-level functions (**Fig. 20**). Diagonal chopping exercises should be performed to facilitate upper body control over a stable lower extremity base.

Initial plyometric movements can be initiated during the later parts of this phase. Initially, small range-of-motion rapid movements, such as quick steps onto a box in the forward and lateral directions are useful in preparing a patient for larger motion hopping or jumping exercises. Progression to modified broad jumps, lateral hops, and single-leg hops can be advanced as tolerated during this phase to assist in neuro-muscular control of both the concentric and eccentric activation phases of explosive

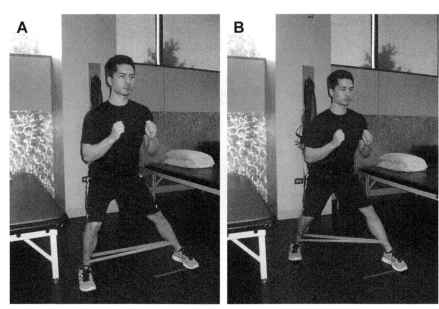

Fig. 20. (*A*) Resistance band standing and (*B*) stepping.

movement. Any increase or change in symptoms may indicate that the patient does not have the foundational muscle strength, endurance, or neuromuscular control for the demand of the exercise; therefore, training should be modified until symptoms subside.

If running is a goal after hip arthroscopy, appropriate running progression exercises should be initiated during this phase.[30] Patients must demonstrate an adequate degree of muscle strength, endurance, and activation patterning to prevent irritation secondary to overuse. Previous investigators have recommended that patients pass assessment that incorporates repeated double-leg squats, step-down, and manual hip abductor strength test prior to the initiation of a running program.[2] Other aspects of previously published return-to-sport tests, such as resisted single-leg squats and lateral agility, may be useful to evaluate sustained movement control and muscle endurance prior to initiating a return-to-running program.[4,13] Patients should be monitored closely during a return-to-run progression and it is recommended that the movement variable of speed should be progressed last.[30]

Phase 4 Neuromuscular Control Exercises

Neuromuscular control exercises in this phase involve high demand training that must focus on speed, agility, power, and skill. The movement patterns are ones performed in sports and occupations that require a high degree of manual labor. Therefore, often an individual's functional demands do not require progression into this final phase of rehabilitation. Because the intensity of the activity performed in this phase increases considerably, it is important to gradually introduce exercises. Initially, variables should be manipulated one at a time to avoid soft tissue irritation secondary to overload.[2] Functional testing may be useful during this phase to monitor progress to help determine when an unrestricted return to high-level activity is appropriate.[31]

Sport-specific and high-demand activities require a great deal of control; therefore, all aspects of movement must be incorporated into a rehabilitation program.

High-velocity and low-velocity movements under load should be advanced to develop muscle strength and power throughout the necessary range of motion.[2,30] Olympic lifting exercises are useful to improve the rate of force development and movement sequencing for high-level activities. Plyometric exercises, such as countermovement jumps or box jumps, can assist with rate of force development and enhance the use of the stretch-shortening cycle.[2,30] Agility exercises, such as cutting, sprinting, and decelerating, should be progressed slowly to the level of sport-specific demand.[13] Skills can be improved through repetition because this assists in patterning the neuromuscular system to improve movement efficiency. The physician, physical therapists, athletic trainers, and coaches must clearly communicate as an athlete transitions to practice and competition. Previous investigators have advised incorporating rest days as athletes return to sports to prevent irritation or reinjury.[2]

SUMMARY

Adequate control of movement is essential for patients to return to unrestricted function after hip arthroscopic surgery. Mobility, muscle performance and stability, and neuromuscular control are vital aspects commonly addressed in rehabilitation to help re-establish control of movement for function. Initial joint protection is a hallmark for all patients after hip arthroscopy to prevent intra-articular and extra-articular soft tissue irritation. Initial mobility exercises should focus on restoration of motion, with these exercises progressed to restore terminal ranges for patients' desired function. Muscle performance and stability exercises should begin with submaximal muscle activations and be transitioned to exercises that involve cocontraction to promote stability for activity of daily living function. Muscle performance and stability exercises should be progressed to incorporate increasing loads to advance demand for higher-level function. Initial neuromuscular control exercises initially should target aberrant movements that may lead to undue stress on healing tissues. As a patient progresses, neuromuscular control exercises are advanced to re-establish coordination and timing of movement for higher-level functions. It is essential to tailor the exercises of each phase to patients' specific demands to prevent soft tissue injury associated with overuse or overload. Each phase of rehabilitation should be closely monitored so that patients are not advanced too quickly, which can lead to setbacks and delays in return to normal function.

REFERENCES

1. Bozic KJ, Chan V, Valone FH, et al. Trends in hip arthroscopy utilization in the united states. J Arthroplasty 2013;28(8):140–3.

2. Edelstein J, Ranawat A, Enseki KR, et al. Post-operative guidelines following hip arthroscopy. Curr Rev Musculoskelet Med 2012;5(1):15–23.

3. Malloy P, Malloy M, Draovitch P. Guidelines and pitfalls for the rehabilitation following hip arthroscopy. Curr Rev Musculoskelet Med 2013;6(3):235–41.

4. Wahoff M, Dischiavi S, Hodge J, et al. Rehabilitation after labral repair and femoroacetabular decompression: criteria-based progression through the return to sport phase. Int J Sports Phys Ther 2014;9(6):813.

5. Cheatham SW, Kolber MJ. Rehabilitation after hip arthroscopy and labral repair in a high school football athlete. Int J Sports Phys Ther 2012;7(2):173–84.

6. Cheatham SW, Enseki KR, Kolber MJ. Post-operative rehabilitation after hip arthroscopy: a search for the evidence. J Sport Rehabil 2014;24(4):413–8.

7. Cheatham SW, Kolber MJ. Rehabilitation after hip arthroscopy and labral repair in a high school football athlete: a 3.6 year follow-up with insight into potential risk factors. Int J Sports Phys Ther 2015;10(4):530.

8. Grzybowski JS, Malloy P, Stegemann C, et al. Rehabilitation following hip arthroscopy-A systematic review. Front Surg 2015;2:21.

9. LeBeau RT, Nho SJ. The use of manual therapy Post–Hip arthroscopy when an exercise-based therapy approach has failed: a case report. J Orthop Sports Phys Ther 2014;44(9):712–21.

10. Enseki KR, Kohlrieser D. Rehabilitation following hip arthroscopy: an evolving process. Int J Sports Phys Ther 2014;9(6):765.

11. Spencer-Gardner L, Eischen JJ, Levy BA, et al. A comprehensive five-phase rehabilitation programme after hip arthroscopy for femoroacetabular impingement. Knee Surg Sports Traumatol Arthrosc 2014;22(4):848–59.

12. Enseki KR, Martin RL, Draovitch P, et al. The hip joint: arthroscopic procedures and postoperative rehabilitation. J Orthop Sports Phys Ther 2006;36(7):516–25.

13. Wahoff M, Ryan M. Rehabilitation after hip femoroacetabular impingement arthroscopy. Clin Sports Med 2011;30(2):463–82.

14. Buckwalter JA, Brown TD. Joint injury, repair, and remodeling: roles in post-traumatic osteoarthritis. Clin Orthop 2004;423:7–16.

15. Neumann DA. Biomechanical analysis of selected principles of hip joint protection. Arthritis Rheum 1989;2(4):146–55.

16. Philippon MJ, Ejnisman L, Ellis HB, et al. Outcomes 2 to 5 years following hip arthroscopy for femoroacetabular impingement in the patient aged 11 to 16 years. Arthroscopy 2012;28(9):1255–61.

17. Byrd JT, Jones KS. Adhesive capsulitis of the hip. Arthroscopy 2006;22(1):89–94.

18. Willimon SC, Briggs KK, Philippon MJ. Intra-articular adhesions following hip arthroscopy: a risk factor analysis. Knee Surg Sports Traumatol Arthrosc 2014; 22(4):822–5.

19. Freeman S, Mascia A, McGill S. Arthrogenic neuromusculature inhibition: a foundational investigation of existence in the hip joint. Clin Biomech 2013;28(2): 171–7.

20. Philippon MJ, Decker MJ, Giphart JE, et al. Rehabilitation exercise progression for the gluteus medius muscle with consideration for iliopsoas tendinitis: an in vivo electromyography study. Am J Sports Med 2011;39(8):1777–85.

21. Lewis CL, Sahrmann SA, Moran DW. Anterior hip joint force increases with hip extension, decreased gluteal force, or decreased iliopsoas force. J Biomech 2007;40(16):3725–31.

22. Anderson FC, Pandy MG. Individual muscle contributions to support in normal walking. Gait Posture 2003;17(2):159–69.

23. van der Krogt MM, Delp SL, Schwartz MH. How robust is human gait to muscle weakness? Gait Posture 2012;36(1):113–9.

24. Ekstrom RA, Donatelli RA, Carp KC. Electromyographic analysis of core trunk, hip, and thigh muscles during 9 rehabilitation exercises. J Orthop Sports Phys Ther 2007;37(12):754–62.

25. Escamilla RF, Lewis C, Bell D, et al. Core muscle activation during swiss ball and traditional abdominal exercises. J Orthop Sports Phys Ther 2010;40(5):265–76.

26. Knuttgen HG, Kraemer WJ. Terminology and measurement in exercise performance. J Strength Cond Res 1987;1(1):1–10.

27. Lamontagne M, Kennedy MJ, Beaulé PE. The effect of cam FAI on hip and pelvic motion during maximum squat. Clin Orthop 2009;467(3):645–50.

28. Lamontagne M, Brisson N, Kennedy MJ, et al. Preoperative and postoperative lower-extremity joint and pelvic kinematics during maximal squatting of patients with cam femoro-acetabular impingement. J Bone Joint Surg Am 2011; 93(Suppl 2):40–5.
29. Rylander J, Shu B, Favre J, et al. Functional testing provides unique insights into the pathomechanics of femoroacetabular impingement and an objective basis for evaluating treatment outcome. J Orthop Res 2013;31(9):1461–8.
30. Draovitch P, Maschi RA, Hettler J. Return to sport following hip injury. Curr Rev Musculoskelet Med 2012;5(1):9–14.
31. Manske R, Reiman M. Functional performance testing for power and return to sports. Sports Health 2013;5(3):244–50.

Index

Note: Page numbers of article titles are in **boldface** type.

Clin Sports Med 35 (2016) 523–528
http://dx.doi.org/10.1016/S0278-5919(16)30035-7
0278-5919/16/$ – see front matter

sportsmed.theclinics.com

Printed and bound by CPI Group (UK) Ltd, Croydon, CR0 4YY

08/05/2025

01864686-0001